DREXEL UNIVERSITY
HEALTH SCIENCES LIBRARIES
QUEEN LANE LIBRARY

Patient Encou...

The Ob...ics
and Gynecology
Work-Up

Rajiv B. Gala, MD
Residency Program Director
Department of Obstetrics and Gynecology
Ochsner Clinic Foundation
New Orleans, Louisiana

Series Editor
Alfa O. Diallo, MD, MPH
Department of Medicine
The Johns Hopkins Hospital
Baltimore, Maryland

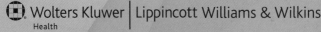

Wolters Kluwer | Lippincott Williams & Wilkins
Health

Philadelphia • Baltimore • New York • London
Buenos Aires • Hong Kong • Sydney • Tokyo

Acquisitions Editor: Susan Rhyner
Product Manager: Stacey L. Sebring
Marketing Manager: Christen Melcher
Compositor: Aptara, Inc.

**WP
39
P298
2010**

Copyright © 2010 Lippincott Williams & Wilkins
351 West Camden Street
Baltimore, Maryland 21201-2436 USA
530 Walnut Street
Philadelphia, PA 19106

All rights reserved. This book is protected by copyright. No part of this book may be reproduced in any form or by any means, including photocopying, or utilized by any information storage and retrieval system without written permission from the copyright owner.

The publisher is not responsible (as a matter of product liability, negligence or otherwise) for any injury resulting from any material contained herein. This publication contains information relating to general principles of medical care which should not be construed as specific instructions for individual patients. Manufacturers' product information and package inserts should be reviewed for current information, including contraindications, dosages and precautions.

Printed in China

Library of Congress Cataloging-in-Publication Data

Patient encounters. The obstetrics and gynecology work-up / editor,
Rajiv B. Gala.
     p. ; cm.
  Includes bibliographical references and index.
  ISBN 978-0-7817-9398-8 (alk. paper)
  1. Obstetrics—Handbooks, manuals, etc. 2. Gynecology—Handbooks,
manuals, etc. 3. Clinical clerkship—Handbooks, manuals, etc. I. Gala,
Rajiv B. II. Title: Obstetrics and gynecology work-up.
  [DNLM: 1. Genital Diseases, Female—Handbooks. 2. Obstetrics—
Handbooks. 3. Pregnancy Complications—Handbooks.   WP 39
P298 2010]
  RG110.P38 2010
  618—dc22

                                                         2009035837

The publishers have made every effort to trace the copyright holders for borrowed material. If they have inadvertently overlooked any, they will be pleased to make the necessary arrangements at the first opportunity.

We'd like to hear from you! If you have comments or suggestions regarding this Lippincott Williams & Wilkins title, please contact us at the appropriate customer service number listed below, or send correspondence to **book_comments@lww.com.** If possible, please remember to include your mailing address, phone number, and a reference to the book title and author in your message. To purchase additional copies of this book call our customer service department at **(800) 638-3030** or fax orders to **(301) 824-7390.** International customers should call **(301) 714-2324.**

CCS1009

Contributing Authors

Sunil Balgobin, MD
Assistant Professor
Department of Obstetrics and
  Gynecology
University of Texas Southwestern
  Medical Center
Faculty
Department of Obstetrics and
  Gynecology
Parkland Health and Hospital System
Dallas, Texas

Victor E. Beshay, MD
Assistant Professor
Department of Obstetrics and
  Gynecology
REI Division
University of Texas Southwestern
  Medical Center
Dallas, Texas

April T. Bleich, MD
Maternal Fetal Medicine Fellow
Department of Obstetrics and
  Gynecology
University of Texas Southwestern
  Medical Center
Dallas, Texas

Justin Brewer, MD
Resident Physician
Department of Obstetrics and
  Gynecology
University of Mississippi School of
  Medicine
Jackson, Mississippi

Cynthia A. Brincat, MD, PhD
Female Pelvic Medicine and
  Reconstructive Surgery Fellow
Department of Obstetrics and
  Gynecology
University of Michigan
Ann Arbor, Michigan

Elena S. Díaz, MD
Resident Physician
Department of Obstetrics and
  Gynecology
University of Texas Southwestern
  Medical Center
Parkland Memorial Hospital
Dallas, Texas

Ravi Gada, MD
Division of Reproductive
  Endocrinology and Infertility
Department of Obstetrics and
  Gynecology
Mayo Clinic
Rochester, Minnesota

Rajiv B. Gala, MD
Residency Program Director
Department of Obstetrics and
  Gynecology
Ochsner Clinic Foundation
New Orleans, Louisiana

Veronica C. Gillispie, MD
Staff Physician
Department of Obstetrics and
  Gynecology
Ochsner Clinic Foundation
New Orleans, Louisiana

Aaron Gingrich, MD
University of Texas Southwestern
  Medical School
Dallas, Texas

Cherine A. Hamid, MD
Assistant Professor
Department of Obstetrics and
   Gynecology
University of Texas Southwestern
   Medical Center
Dallas, Texas

Amaryllis Hays, MD
Resident Physician
Department of Obstetrics and
   Gynecology
University of Texas Southwestern
   Medical Center
Dallas, Texas

Meadow Maze Good, DO
Resident Physician
Department of Obstetrics and
   Gynecology
University of Texas Southwestern
   Medical Center
Parkland Memorial Hospital
Dallas, Texas

Jennifer Griffin, MD
Instructor
Department of Obstetrics and
   Gynecology
University of Nebraska Medical Center
Omaha, Nebraska

Stacey L. Holman, MD
Clinical Instructor
Department of Obstetrics and
   Gynecology
Louisiana State University
Health Sciences Center
New Orleans, Louisiana

Emily Brewer Johnson, DO
Resident Physician
Department of Obstetrics and
   Gynecology
University of Mississippi Medical
   Center
Jackson, Mississippi

Jennifer Mendillo Keller, MD, MPH
Assistant Professor
Department of Obstetrics and
   Gynecology
The George Washington University
Washington, D.C.

Jonathan Kim, MD
Resident Physician
Department of Obstetrics and
   Gynecology
University of Texas Southwestern
   Medical Center
Dallas, Texas

Louise P. King, MD, JD
Resident Physician
Department of Obstetrics and
   Gynecology
University of Texas Southwestern
   Medical Center
Parkland Memorial Hospital
Dallas, Texas

Phyllis E. Lawani, MD
Resident Physician
Department of Obstetrics and
   Gynecology
University of Texas Southwestern
   Medical Center
Parkland Memorial Hospital
Dallas, Texas

Dennis D. Mauricio, MD
Resident Physician
Department of Obstetrics and
   Gynecology
University of Buffalo-SUNY
Buffalo, New York

David D. Rahn, MD, FACOG
Assistant Professor, Female Pelvic
    Medicine & Reconstructive
    Surgery
Department of Obstetrics and
    Gynecology
University of Texas Southwestern
    Medical Center
Dallas, Texas

Tanisha Silas, MD
Resident
Department of Obstetrics and
    Gynecology
University of Texas Southwestern
    Medical Center
Parkland Memorial Hospital
Dallas, Texas

Jose Tiran-Saucedo, MD
Professor
Department of Maternal Fetal Medicine
    Institute/CGOMSA
Universidad de Monterrey (UDEM)
Medical Director
Department of Clinical Services and
    Research
Mexican Institute of Infectious Diseases in
    Obstetrics and Gynecology (IMIGO)
Monterrey, Neuvo Leon, Mexico

Kristy K. Ward, MD
Resident Physician
Department of Obstetrics and
    Gynecology
University of Texas Medical Branch at
    Galveston
Galveston, Texas

Series Reviewers

Janeen Arbuckle
University of Oklahoma Health
  Sciences Center

Teresa Cabezas
Florida State University College of
  Medicine

Peggy Constant
Long Island Jewish Medical Center

Ashwini Sagar Davison, MD
Johns Hopkins Hospital

Melissa Garber
University of Kansas School of Medicine

Emily Godlewski
University of Toledo College of Medicine

Kendra D. Hayslett, MD
Nashville Metro General Hospital

Matthew G. Hoyt, DO
Eglin Hospital

Zi Yang Jiang
University of Illinois at Chicago

Jay Kalawadia
Northwestern University, Feinberg
  School of Medicine

Cindy Lee
Midwestern University of Arizona
  College of Medicine

Lynne Matsuoka
Keck School of Medicine, University of
  Southern California

**Elizabeth Marie Salisbury Afshar,
MD**
Illinois Masonic Medical Center

Robert W. Sedlacek, MD
Rush University
Rush Copley Medical Center

Jessica Stine
University of Miami

T. Renee Williams
Meharry Medical College

Nathan Zilbert
New York University

Preface

The *Patient Encounters* series has been developed to provide a concise review of patient assessment and management. Each book in this series is organized logically and provides medical students with specialty-specific steps for managing patient care. The goal of this series is to remove the focus from "acing the shelf" to a focus on helping medical students become good doctors.

The books in this series provide a specialty-specific, step-by-step guide for managing a patient by candidly addressing, in a very practical fashion, a new clinical clerk's anxiety as well as hunger for learning. Each title within this series is a companion guide that candidly cuts to need-to-know info, directing medical students to what they need to do in each step of the patient encounter.

The books in this series discuss patient care from an overview of the disease or disorder, with brief pathophysiology information presented as necessary to support optimal patient assessment and care. It includes specific information that will help medical students from the point of reviewing the patient's chart to walking into the room and assessing the stability of the patient, including potential life threats. Each book then addresses acute management and workup, directing the student through the diagnosis, treatment, extended inhospital management, and discharge goals and outpatient care.

Each title provides students with the rationale for ordering appropriate diagnostic studies and allows clinical decision making that is consistent with the patient's disposition. The books provide an extended view of patient care so that the medical student can propose a well-informed choice of diagnostic studies and interventions when presenting his or her case to house staff and faculty.

The books use algorithms, tables, figures, icons, and a stylized design to support concise and easy-to-find patient management information. They also provide diagnosis-based, evidence-based information that includes peer-reviewed journal references.

Feedback from student reviewers gives high praise to this new series. Each of these new books was developed to provide practical information and to address the basics needed during a particular clinical rotation:

Patient Encounters: The Inpatient Pediatrics Work-Up
Patient Encounters: The Neurology and Psychiatry Work-Up
Patient Encounters: The Internal Medicine Work-Up

How to Use This Book

Patient Encounters: The Obstetrics and Gynecology Work-Up provides you with a concise, organized review of the most important patient assessment and management in obstetrics and gynecology. This book is designed for you to quickly and efficiently review and enhance the knowledge you need to effectively manage patient care.

This book can help you ease the transition from the basic sciences to clinical medicine by providing you with a practical "how-to" guide for approaching a patient, including:

- Identifying pertinent positives and negatives in the patient history and physical exam
- Determining how to work up a patient by addressing pertinent diagnostic studies and procedures
- Explaining the rationale for clinical decision making

The 30 chapters in this text are divided into 6 sections that are supplemented with 3 appendices. Each chapter features essential information related to patient assessment and management, supplemented with patient case studies that provide you with the opportunity to apply patient care principles and management goals to patient cases that are specific to each chapter's topic.

This book, as with all the books in the series, includes common features that will allow you to glean necessary information quickly and easily:

- **The Patient Encounter:** Each chapter begins with a patient case study that is followed up on at several intervals throughout the chapter. The patient encounter allows you the opportunity to see some of the common signs and symptoms with which a patient may present.
- **Overview:** This section provides an introduction to the chapter topic and includes the definition, epidemiology, and etiology of the disease or disorder. Brief pathophysiology information is included to support optimal patient assessment and care.
- **Acute Management and Workup:** This section includes the key information that you need to obtain in order to provide excellent patient care, addressing first what you need to do within the first 15 minutes through the first few hours. Topics include the initial assessment, admission criteria and level of care criteria, the patient history, the physical examination, labs and imaging to consider, and key treatment information.
- **Extended Inhospital Management:** This section provides information that you need to know when a patient needs extended inhospital management.

- **Disposition:** In this section, you will find the key discharge goals and out-patient care related to a patient with the specific condition or disorder addressed in the chapter.
- **What You Need to Remember:** This feature is a bulleted list of key points that are most helpful to remember about the chapter topic.
- **Suggested Readings:** Each chapter provides diagnosis- and evidence-based peer-reviewed journal references.
- **Clinical Pearl:** This feature presents clinical tips, statistics, or findings that will help you understand the patient's clinical presentation or help you better address diagnosis and management.

In addition to the features noted above, this text contains tables, line drawings, and photographs to supplement your learning.

I hope this text improves your knowledge of obstetrics and gynecology, allowing you to feel confident that you're providing quality patient care. The ultimate goal of this book is to better prepare you to provide effective care to patients who you will encounter in your medical career.

Rajiv B. Gala, MD
Residency Program Director
Department of Obstetrics and Gynecology
Ochsner Clinic Foundation
New Orleans, Louisiana

Contents

Preconception Counseling

THE PATIENT ENCOUNTER

A 36-year-old woman (G0) presents to your office for her annual gynecologic exam. She mentions to you that she is recently engaged and interested in starting a family in the next 6 months. She would like to know more about what she should do to optimize her chances of having a healthy pregnancy.

OVERVIEW

Definition

There is a misconception that prenatal care begins when a woman is pregnant. In reality, prenatal care begins with preconception counseling. This is the time to evaluate a woman's risk to herself and to her fetus. This also allows the ability to anticipate and prevent possible complications to the pregnancy.

Epidemiology

During each gynecology visit with patients of childbearing age, a discussion regarding their plans for pregnancy should take place. This allows you to discuss contraception with those who want to prevent pregnancy, thereby lowering the rate of unplanned pregnancies. It is estimated that in 2001, the rate of unplanned pregnancies was 49% (1). This rate is unchanged from 1994. It is the goal of *Healthy People 2010* that the rate of unintended pregnancies be decreased to 30% by the year 2010.

CLINICAL PEARL

Pregnancies are unplanned in approximately 49% of all cases.

ACUTE MANAGEMENT AND WORKUP

For those who are interested in conceiving, a risk assessment should be performed. This is done by gathering a detailed history, performing a physical exam, and performing various laboratory tests. From this information, you can best counsel the patient regarding the optimal time for pregnancy to occur to achieve the best maternal and fetal outcome.

History

The first obstetric visit is an excellent opportunity for you to empower your patient with tools to improve her overall health. During the reproductive years of a woman's life, pregnancy may be the only reason your patient engages in routine health care. A complete history must include the following: past medical history, past obstetric history, past surgical history, family history, and social history.

Past Medical History

Poor control of various medical problems not only causes complications for a pregnancy but can prevent conception all together. Poor control of chronic diseases such as hypothyroidism or diabetes can prevent ovulation. Patients should have optimal control of their chronic diseases prior to conceiving. Two of the most encountered chronic conditions in women of childbearing age are hypertension and diabetes.

Chronic hypertension is one of the most common medical conditions that complicates pregnancy. Patients with chronic hypertension are at increased risk for superimposed pre-eclampsia, placental abruption, intrauterine growth restriction, and other complications. Chronic hypertension is defined as a systolic blood pressure of ≥ 140 mm Hg and a diastolic blood pressure of ≥ 90 mm Hg before 20 weeks gestational age on two occasions at least 4 hours apart (2). Chronic hypertension can further be divided into mild and severe chronic hypertension. Mild chronic hypertension is defined as a blood pressure $\geq 140/90$ mm Hg, while severe chronic hypertension is defined as a blood pressure $\geq 180/110$ mm Hg (Table 1-1).

In the preconception evaluation of chronic hypertension, the severity of the hypertension must be assessed. Patients who have experienced end-organ damage are at increased risk of worsening damage during pregnancy and should be aware of this risk.

TABLE 1-1
Mild and Severe Chronic Hypertension in Pregnancy

Type of Chronic Hypertension	Systolic Pressure (mm Hg)	Diastolic Pressure (mm Hg)
Mild	≥ 140	≥ 90
Severe	≥ 180	≥ 110

There should also be an assessment of the antihypertensive medications your patient takes to minimize exposure to potential teratogens. For example, the use of angiotensin-converting enzyme inhibitors in the second and third trimesters has been shown to cause oligohydramnios, fetal limb abnormalities, and craniofacial abnormalities (3). Patients should be switched to an antihypertensive medication that is safe in pregnancy. Methyldopa is the most widely studied medication for long-term fetal and maternal safety. The target blood pressure for patients with chronic hypertension is 150/90 mm Hg. Antihypertensive medications should be given if blood pressures are consistently >160/110 mm Hg. Lowering the blood pressure too much can be as detrimental as a persistently elevated blood pressure. Both hypotension and severe hypertension can lead to intrauterine growth restriction due to decreased uteroplacental perfusion.

Diabetes mellitus is another common chronic medical condition that can complicate pregnancy. Chronic diabetes can be divided into type I or type II. Type I diabetes is a chronic metabolic disorder in which there is lack of insulin production. In type II diabetes, while insulin is produced, it is insufficient relative to the amount of glucose present. For either condition, euglycemia is paramount during pregnancy.

Poor control of diabetes early in gestation can result in spontaneous abortion. Those gestations that do continue are at increased risk for several fetal anomalies. Rare in its occurrence, the congenital anomaly most characteristic of diabetes is sacral agenesis. Cardiac and CNS malformations are much more common. Ventral septal defects are increased 5- and CNS malformations such as anencephaly and open spina bifida are increased 10-fold (2). These defects occur during the first 7 weeks of gestation.

Fetal growth can also be affected by poor glycemic control. This can be in the form of macrosomia or intrauterine growth restriction. Macrosomia is defined as a fetal weight of ≥4,500 g for a fetus born to a diabetic mother. In macrosomia, maternal hyperglycemia causes fetal hyperinsulinemia, resulting in excessive fetal growth. This can also cause neonatal hypoglycemia after delivery. Intrauterine growth restriction results from uteroplacental insufficiency due to vascular damage as a result of poor glucose control.

There are many other complications associated with the poor control of diabetes. One of these is fetal respiratory distress syndrome, which results from the decreased production of surfactant as a result of poor glycemic control. Stillbirth is also increased for women with poorly controlled diabetes. Most often this occurs after 36 weeks of gestation. Although not well understood, the presumed mechanism of action is thought to be due to vascular damage. Because anomalies can begin to occur as early as 7 weeks gestational age, preconception counseling to ensure euglycemia is necessary for diabetic women.

CLINICAL PEARL

The prepregnancy target for your patient's hemoglobin A1C is 6% (4).

Included in the medical history is any history of psychiatric disorders. Patients with a history of major depressive disorder are at increased risk for postpartum depression. These patients should be watched closely during the antepartum period for development of signs of worsening depression.

Past Obstetric History

The patient's previous obstetric history consists of the number of pregnancies and the outcome of those pregnancies. Patients with recurrent spontaneous abortions should be evaluated for thrombophilias such as antiphospholipid antibody syndrome, and for parental genetic karyotyping. Approximately 50% of spontaneous abortions in the first trimester are due to chromosomal abnormalities (2). Patients with a history of preterm delivery have an increased risk of preterm delivery with subsequent pregnancies.

Past Surgical History

Your patient's surgical history should also be obtained. Patients with a history of uterine surgery, such as a myomectomy, that involves entry into the uterine cavity are counseled against having a vaginal delivery because of the increased risk of uterine rupture. Patients with a previous low transverse cesarean section may attempt a vaginal birth after cesarean section but they must be aware of the potential risk of uterine rupture.

Family History

Family history is an integral part of preconception counseling. Questions should be targeted to elicit any family history of Down syndrome, neural tube defects, mental retardation, and other birth defects. The family history should also include any history of inherited diseases such as cystic fibrosis, sickle cell disease, and Huntington chorea. A family history that is significant for any of these findings may necessitate additional interventions, such as genetic testing.

Social History

The social history addresses socioeconomic status, occupational risk factors, nutrition status, and abuse. Low socioeconomic status has been associated with preterm delivery, low birth weight, poor nutritional status, and substance abuse.

During preconception counseling, the physician should address possible hazards that are related to the patient's occupation. This may vary from

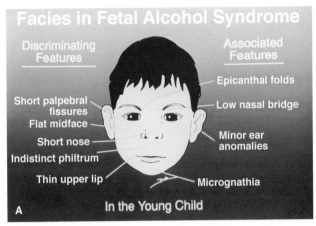

FIGURE 1-1: Characteristics of a child with fetal alcohol syndrome.

exposure to different chemicals to physical risks that may negatively affect the pregnancy. The patient should engage her employer to make any necessary adjustments to her job description to ensure a healthy pregnancy.

All forms of abuse negatively affect pregnancy, including the use of tobacco, alcohol, and drugs, and/or violence. Tobacco abuse has been shown to increase the risk of spontaneous abortion, infants that are small for gestational age, and sudden infant death syndrome. There are several tools, such as medications, nicotine patches, and exercise, to assist those women who are motivated to stop smoking.

Alcohol abuse can lead to a disorder known as "fetal alcohol syndrome" (Fig. 1-1). Infants with fetal alcohol syndrome often suffer from growth retardation, mental retardation, and characteristic facial features such as small palpebral fissures, epicanthic folds, a flattened nasal bridge, and low-set ears (2) The exact amount of alcohol necessary to cause these detrimental side effects is not known. When addressing a patient's alcohol assumption, the "CAGE" questions can be helpful:

1. Have you ever tried to **CUT** down on your drinking?
2. Do you get **ANGRY** when someone asks you about the amount you drink?
3. Do you ever feel **GUILTY** about the amount of alcohol you drink?
4. Do you ever need an **EYEOPENER** in the morning?

During preconception counseling, the physician should inquire about substance abuse. Patients who are abusing drugs may not readily admit to doing so. Physicians must then hone in to the signs of drug abuse, such as vague physical complaints (headaches, loss of appetite, dizziness, trouble in personal relationships). A brief intervention should follow the "five As":

1. **Ask** about drug abuse
2. **Assess** if abuse exists
3. **Advise** patients to discontinue drug use
4. **Assist** patients in quitting the abuse
5. **Arrange** for follow-up of the intervention (5)

The possibility of domestic abuse should also be addressed during preconception counseling. Continued physical abuse during pregnancy can result in injury or death to the mother and/or the fetus. Patients often do not reveal they are in an abusive relationship and have a tendency to return to their abuser. If abuse is suspected, you should ensure that the patient is in a safe environment and encourage the patient to develop a plan of escape from her abuser (5).

Medications

When a patient is seen for preconception counseling, a list of active medications should be reviewed. Medications that are contraindicated in pregnancy because of teratogenicity should be stopped immediately. Over-the-counter medications should be avoided unless approved by the patient's physician. All prenatal vitamins contain at least the minimum U.S. Recommended Daily Allowance of folic acid (0.4 mg) for neural tube defect prevention. If your patient has a history of an infant born with a neural tube defect, the Centers for Disease Control and American College of Obstetricians and Gynecologists recommend 4 mg of folic acid per day (6).

CLINICAL PEARL

Taking 0.4 mg of folic acid during the preconception period and throughout the first trimester could prevent nearly half of all neural tube defects in the United States (7). Patients with a history of an infant with a neural tube defect should increase their folic acid intake to 4 mg daily.

Physical Examination

Preconception counseling should include a complete physical exam. This should include documentation of the patient's prepregnancy weight, as well as her current vital signs, weight, and height. This information will assist in determining if proper weight gain is achieved throughout the pregnancy. The physical exam should continue with a breast, cardiac, lung, abdominal, and pelvic exam. A Papanicolaou smear as well as culture for gonorrhea and chlamydia should be obtained during the pelvic exam.

Laboratory Evaluations

Laboratory evaluations are as important as the physical exam. A complete blood count should be obtained to evaluate for anemia. The blood type, Rh status, and antibody screen can alert you to the risk of subsequent isoimmunization problems. If a patient is rubella nonimmune, the vaccine can be given but conception should be deferred for at least 3 months. In addition to gonorrhea and chlamydia cultures that are obtained during the pelvic exam, patients should be tested for human immunodeficiency virus, hepatitis B, and syphilis. Urine should be tested for infection, as well as glucose and protein levels.

 WHAT YOU NEED TO REMEMBER

- Prenatal care begins with preconception counseling. During each gynecologic visit with patients of childbearing age, you should discuss their plans for pregnancy.
- For those interested in conceiving, an assessment should take place that involves gathering a detailed history, performing a physical exam, and obtaining various laboratory values.
- Poor control of various medical problems not only causes complications for a pregnancy but can prevent conception all together. Two of the most encountered chronic conditions in women of childbearing age are hypertension and diabetes.
- The surgical history can impact the route of delivery.
- Family history should be obtained regarding the presence of Down syndrome, neural tube defects, mental retardation, and other birth defects.
- The U.S. Recommended Daily Allowance of folic acid for pregnant women is 0.4 mg every day to prevent neural tube defects. Women with a history of an infant born with a neural tube defect should increase their folic acid intake to 4 mg every day.

REFERENCES

1. Finer LB, Henshaw SK. Disparities in the rates of unintended pregnancy in the United States, 1994 and 2001. *Perspect Sex Reprod Health*. 2006;38:90–96.
2. Gabbe S, Niebyl JR, Simpson JL. *Obstetrics: Normal and Problem Pregnancies*. 4th ed. New York, NY: Churchill Livingstone; 2002.

3. Briggs GG, Freeman RK, Yaffe, SJ. *Drugs in Pregnancy and Lactation.* 7th ed. Philadelphia, PA: Lippincott Williams & Wilkins; 2005.
4. American College of Obstetricians and Gynecologists. ACOG practice bulletin number 60: March 2005. Pregestational diabetes mellitus. Clinical management guidelines for obstetricians-gynecologists. *Obstet Gynecol.* 2005;105(3):675–685.
5. American College of Obstetrics and Gynecologists. *Special Issues in Women's Health.* Washington, DC: Author; 2005.
6. Centers for Disease Control and Prevention. Recommendations for the use of folic acid to reduce the number of cases of spina bifida and other neural tube defects. *MMWR Morb Mortal Wkly Rep.* 1992;41.
7. Centers for Disease Control and Prevention. Knowledge and use of folic acid by women of childbearing age—United States 1995–1998. *MMWR Morb Mortal Wkly Rep.* 1999;48(16):325–327.

Labor and Delivery

THE PATIENT ENCOUNTER

At 0800, you are paged by the nurse to evaluate a woman who "thinks she's in labor." She is a 24-year-old woman who is 39 weeks pregnant (G1P0). She reports feeling strong contractions since midnight, which are now about 3 to 4 minutes apart. You can tell she is uncomfortable; she is breathing heavily with each contraction. She states she has not had any bleeding or leaking of fluid. In review of her prenatal record, her pregnancy has been uncomplicated.

OVERVIEW

Definition

Labor, in an obstetrical sense, is regular, progressively intense contractions that cause dilation and effacement of the cervix, ultimately leading to delivery of the infant and placenta. Labor is diagnosed clinically when a woman presents with contractions, and change in the cervix is documented. Spontaneous labor will generally occur at term, which is defined as the period between 36 and 41 completed weeks of pregnancy. If labor occurs prior to 36 completed weeks, it is considered preterm labor.

Normal labor can be divided into four stages: (i) clinical onset of labor, (ii) fetal descent and delivery of the baby, (iii) delivery of the placenta and membranes, and (iv) the puerperium. The first stage is further separated into two components: The latent period is the time from the onset of regular uterine contractions to the time in which the cervix begins to change at an accelerated rate. This accelerated (active) phase will occur after the cervix reaches 3 to 5 cm. Therefore, when a woman presents with regular, painful contractions and is found to be 3 to 5 cm dilated, she is generally thought to have reached the threshold for active labor, and is admitted to labor and delivery. The patient enters the second stage of labor once the cervix is completely dilated. During this stage, progressive descent of the fetus through the birth canal should occur. This descent may be aided by the expulsive efforts of the mother. The third stage follows the delivery of the infant, and concludes with delivery of the placenta (1).

Pathophysiology

During the course of labor and delivery, various events may necessitate intervention in this natural process to facilitate or expedite delivery of the infant, including the need for operative delivery in some cases. The events that lead to intervention can be characterized as maternal indications, labor abnormalities, or fetal indications. Maternal indications to expedite delivery occur less frequently, and are addressed under other topics in this book. This chapter will focus on labor abnormalities, but will also include a basic overview of fetal heart rate assessment, which has become the primary means to assess fetal well-being during labor. Electronic fetal heart rate monitoring was performed during only 45% of labors in 1980, but recently used during 85% of labors in the United States in 2002, making it the most commonly performed obstetrical procedure (2). Table 2-1 provides definitions of fetal heart rate patterns with examples illustrated in Figure 2-1.

Spontaneous labor should continue to progress at an appropriate rate; failure to do so may indicate inadequacy of one or more aspects that would predict an inability to accomplish the delivery vaginally. If labor does not progress or progresses at an inappropriately slow rate, these disorders are referred to collectively as *labor dystocia*. For a nulliparous woman, one should expect the cervix to dilate a minimum of 1.2 cm/h during the active phase of labor. For a parous woman, the cervix should dilate at least 1.5 cm/h during the active phase. During the expulsive phase (stage 2), the bony vertex of the fetal head should descend by at least 1 cm/h for a nulliparous woman, and at least 2 cm/h for a parous woman (1). The total length of the second stage should be no more than 1 hour for a parous woman without regional analgesia, 2 hours for a parous woman with regional analgesia or a nulliparous woman without, and 3 hours for a nulliparous woman with regional analgesia (Table 2-2).

Epidemiology

Of the more than 4 million deliveries that occur in the United States each year, approximately 25% of births occur via cesarean section. According to the American College of Obstetricians and Gynecologists, 60% of cesarean deliveries in nulliparous women are due to labor dystocia (3). Approximately 15% are due to fetal distress (4). Another 8% of vaginal births are accomplished by operative vaginal delivery (vacuum or forceps-assisted) for either fetal or labor indications, although the use of these instruments has declined substantially in recent years (5).

Etiology

Failure of labor to progress appropriately may indicate that the fetus cannot pass through the maternal bony pelvis because of relative discordance of size or malposition (frequently referred to as *cephalopelvic disproportion*), or it may indicate that the strength or frequency of uterine contractions is inadequate

TABLE 2-1
Definitions of Fetal Heart Rate Patterns

Pattern	Definition
Baseline	• The mean FHR^a rounded to increments of 5 beats per min during a 10-min segment, excluding: • Periodic or episodic changes • Periods of marked FHR variability • Segments of baseline that differ by more than 25 beats per min • The baseline must be for a minimum of 2 min in any 10-min segment
Baseline variability	• Fluctuations in the FHR of two cycles per min or greater • Variability is visually quantitated as the amplitude of peak-to-trough in beats per min • Absent—amplitude range undetectable • Minimal—amplitude range detectable but 5 beats per min or fewer • Moderate (normal)—amplitude range 6–25 beats per min • Marked—amplitude range >25 beats per min
Acceleration	• A visually apparent increase (onset to peak in <30 sec) in the FHR from the most recently calculated baseline • The duration of an acceleration is defined as the time from the initial change in FHR from the baseline to the return of the FHR to the baseline • At 32 weeks of gestation and beyond, an acceleration has an acme of 15 beats per min or more above baseline, with a duration of ≥15 sec but <2 min • Before 32 weeks of gestation, an acceleration has an acme of 10 beats per min or more above baseline, with a duration of ≥10 sec but <2 min • Prolonged acceleration lasts ≥2 min but <10 min • If an acceleration lasts 10 min or longer, it is a baseline change

(continued)

TABLE 2-1
Definitions of Fetal Heart Rate Patterns (Continued)

Pattern	Definition
Bradycardia	• Baseline FHR <110 beats per min
Early deceleration	• In association with a uterine contraction, a visually apparent, gradual (onset to nadir ≥30 sec) decrease in FHR with return to baseline • Nadir of the deceleration occurs at the same time as the peak of the contraction
Late deceleration	• In association with a uterine contraction, a visually apparent, gradual (onset to nadir ≥30 sec) decrease in FHR with return to baseline • Onset, nadir, and recovery of the deceleration occur after the beginning, peak, and end of the contraction, respectively
Tachycardia	• Baseline FHR >160 beats per min
Variable deceleration	• An abrupt (onset to nadir <30 sec), visually apparent decrease in the FHR below the baseline • The decrease in FHR is ≥15 beats per min, with a duration of ≥15 sec but <2 min
Prolonged deceleration	• Visually apparent decrease in the FHR below the baseline • Deceleration is ≥15 beats per min, lasting ≥2 min but <10 min from onset to return to baseline

*a*FHR, fetal heart rate.
Reprinted from Electronic fetal heart rate monitoring: research guidelines for interpretation, National Institute of Child Health and Human Development Research Planning Workshop, *Am J Obstet Gynecol.* 1997;177:1385–1390, , with permission from Elsevier.

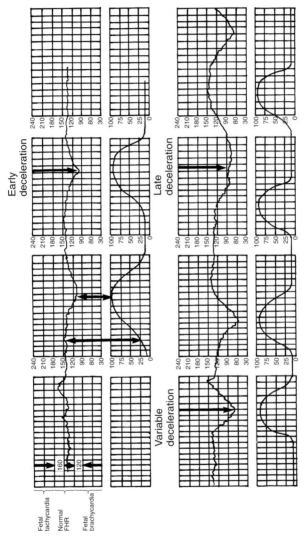

FIGURE 2-1: Fetal heart rate patterns.

TABLE 2-2

Criteria for the Diagnosis of Labor Disorders

Labor Pattern	Nulliparous	Parous
Protraction disorder		
Dilatation	<1.2 cm/h	<1.5 cm/h
Descent	<1.0 cm/h	<2.0 cm/h
Arrest disorder		
No dilatation	>2 h	>2 h
No descent	>1 h	>1 h
Total length of second stage		
Without regional analgesia	2 h	1 h
With regional analgesia	3 h	2 h

to move the fetus through the pelvis. Commonly, more than one factor may contribute to labor dystocia. A mnemonic used to describe these considerations is the "three Ps": (i) the power, (ii) the passenger, and (iii) the pelvis (1).

The Power

The power refers to evaluation of the strength and frequency of uterine contractions. This can be assessed by several means. Most simply, the frequency and strength of contractions can be determined by palpation of the maternal abdomen. A woman in active labor should be having at least three strong contractions every 10 minutes (3). The frequency of contractions can also be determined by external uterine monitoring, called *tocodynamometry*. A more exact assessment of uterine activity can be accomplished by placement of an intrauterine pressure catheter (IUPC). This tool can provide information about both the frequency and strength of contractions. The strength of contractions is determined using Montevideo units, which are calculated by subtracting the baseline uterine pressure from the peak contraction pressure in mm Hg, and adding the total pressures over 10 minutes. Adequate contractions should total 200 Montevideo units or more in 10 minutes.

The Passenger

An estimate of fetal size should be considered for all patients presenting in labor, but is of special significance in situations in which labor is protracted or arrested. This is generally accomplished via Leopold maneuvers, during which you palpate the fetus through the maternal abdomen to estimate size. One should also consider whether risk factors for fetal macrosomia exist, including gestational diabetes, excessive maternal weight gain, maternal obesity, family history of macrosomic infants, and postterm pregnancy. In some cases, ultrasound may be used to estimate fetal weight prior to labor, but one must recognize that ultrasound estimates may be less accurate in the term pregnancy.

In addition to considerations of fetal size, the presentation of the fetus and position of the presenting part may contribute to labor dystocias. The most common position of the fetal vertex at the onset of labor is transverse, which should transition to the occiput pointing anteriorly (OA), or deviated slightly to the left (LOA) or to the right (ROA) during active labor. It is in these positions that the fetus can most easily complete the cardinal movements of labor. If the occiput of the vertex points posteriorly (OP) or remains transverse, this can lead to protraction of labor. Asynclitism, or lateral deflection of the head, can also contribute to labor dystocias.

Although ideally detected at the time of the patient's admission to labor and delivery, malpresentation may be detected during the evaluation of protracted or arrested labor. Presentations such as brow, face, or even breech presentations would be expected to alter the normal time course of labor. Management of these special circumstances will not be covered here, although current standard of care does require cesarean section for most cases of breech presentation in labor.

The Pelvis

An assessment of the maternal pelvis for adequacy should be performed via clinical pelvimetry. This consists of a digital examination in which the following are evaluated: the anteroposterior diameter of the pelvic inlet, the interspinous diameter of the midpelvis, the intertuberous distance of the pelvic outlet, and the pelvic arch. Risk factors for a contracted pelvis may include congenital malformations and a history of pelvic fractures. Radiologic evaluation of pelvic size has been found to be of limited value, and is rarely used. In addition to the bony pelvis, soft tissues can contribute to labor dystocia.

ACUTE MANAGEMENT AND WORKUP

There are two basic questions you must answer when patients acutely present to labor and delivery: (i) Is the fetus term (or preterm), and (ii) is the patient in labor? These answers will help you efficiently make treatment decisions in a busy labor ward.

The First 15 Minutes

When your patient presents to labor and delivery complaining of contractions, the most important question to answer in the first 15 minutes is whether or not she is in active labor. Patients can remain in the latent phase of labor with sporadic contractions for weeks. If fetal well-being is documented, augmentation of labor is recommended only if your patient is full term (greater than 39 weeks) and she has a favorably dilated cervix (>3 cm).

Initial Assessment

A systematic process can be used to assess the patient presenting to labor and delivery with labor-related complaints. This should begin with a detailed history and physical exam, and should include the steps noted in the following sections.

Inquire about Labor-Related Symptoms

The first step is to inquire about labor-related symptoms. Specifically, one should ask when contractions began, how frequently they are occurring, whether they are regularly spaced, and the amount of pain perceived by the patient. The patient in labor will appear uncomfortable, and likely will not be able to carry out a prolonged conversation because of ongoing painful contractions. It is also necessary to inquire about the possible rupture of membranes or bleeding. Some light bleeding is normal in labor as the cervix dilates ("bloody show"), but heavy bleeding should prompt further evaluation.

Monitor Maternal Vital Signs

Maternal vital signs should be obtained at the time of arrival, and abnormalities addressed.

Monitor the Fetal Heart Rate

Electronic fetal heart rate monitoring is generally performed as part of the evaluation process to screen for fetal well-being. The normal baseline fetal heart rate for a term fetus is between 120 and 160 beats per minute. A reassuring fetal heart rate pattern is also characterized by moderate variability and accelerations (Table 2-1). Tocodynamometry is also used to assess the frequency and regularity of contractions.

Review the Prenatal Record

The prenatal record, if available, should be reviewed to identify any risk factors for the patient prior to proceeding with an examination. It is also critical to determine the gestational age at presentation and how it was verified (last menstrual period or ultrasound). If the patient is preterm, this may alter management, including the possible need for tocolysis in a pregnancy earlier than 34 weeks.

Perform a Sterile Speculum Examination of the Cervix

At this point, a cervical exam can be performed. If the patient has complaints of heavy bleeding, a speculum exam should be performed to visually inspect the cervix and vagina. Don't forget to exclude the possibility of placenta previa by ultrasound prior to a digital exam in patients who present with bleeding without prior ultrasound documentation of normal placentation! A speculum exam should also be done to evaluate for rupture of membranes if symptoms exist. If the patient is preterm, then a speculum exam should be done, including visual inspection of the cervix and additional testing that includes a sample for a wet mount, group B streptococcal cultures, fetal fibronectin (if between 24 and 34 weeks of gestation), and gonorrhea/chlamydia cultures.

CLINICAL PEARL

You should always perform a sterile speculum exam before a digital exam of the cervix when you are called to evaluate a pregnant patient complaining of bleeding or leakage of fluid.

Perform a Digital Examination of the Cervix

For routine labor complaints without the above issues, a digital exam of the cervix is generally sufficient. The index and middle finger are inserted into the vagina, and an assessment is made of the dilation and effacement of the cervix. The **dilation** is judged at the level of the internal os by spreading the fingers to assess the diameter. **Effacement** is determined based on the percentage of cervical thinning, assuming the cervix is approximately 4 cm at baseline. For example, if the cervix is approximately 2 cm thick, then it is 50% effaced. The position of the cervix (anterior, midposition, or posterior) can be determined. The cervix of a laboring woman is generally oriented anteriorly. Also, the presentation of the fetus should be documented, as presentations other than occiput may require additional intervention. The **station** of the presenting fetal part should be determined based on the level of the lowest bony part in relation to the ischial spines, measured in centimeters. If the presenting part is above the ischial spines, a negative number is assigned: -1, -2, -3, -4, or -5. (i.e., 1 cm above the ischial spines, and so forth.) The presenting part at the ischial spines is 0 station. When the bony presenting part of the fetal head is at 0 station, it is said to be "engaged." At this level in a vertex presentation, the biparietal diameter of the head will have passed the pelvic inlet. If the presenting part is below the ischial spines (i.e., closer to the introitus), then this is designated as $+1$, $+2$, $+3$, $+4$, or $+5$. The presenting part at $+4$ to $+5$ station is visible at the introitus as it will divide the labia without expulsive efforts (1).

If the patient is having regular, painful contractions and the cervix is found to be 3 to 5 cm dilated, the patient will generally be admitted for presumed active labor management. Bear in mind that not all patients will enter the active phase at 3 cm, so some clinical judgment should be used when making the decision to admit the patient.

If the patient is <3 cm dilated, has intact membranes, documented fetal well-being, and is not having regular, painful contractions, then she is a candidate for ongoing outpatient management. The patient should be educated regarding the symptoms for which she should return, and advised to continue her routine prenatal care until labor ensues.

Admission Criteria and Level of Care Criteria

In general, the patient who is 3 to 5 cm dilated with regular, painful contractions will be admitted for labor. If membranes are ruptured, admission is indicated even if active labor criteria are not met.

Option 1: Stable Condition

The term patient with no major risk factors for labor complications should be admitted for routine labor management. This will generally include placement of an intravenous (IV) line, laboratory testing, monitoring of maternal vital signs every 4 hours at a minimum, and fetal monitoring (1). Tocodynamometry is often done, but not required. An IV access is recommended in case of emergency, but continuous IV fluids need not be administered in the normal laboring woman unless analgesia is being given. Oral intake of solid food should be avoided, and liquids given only sparingly to reduce the risk of aspiration. Examination findings, including cervical exam, presentation of the fetus, estimated fetal weight, and an assessment of clinical adequacy of the pelvis, should be documented on all patients at the time of admission in the medical record! If presentation is in doubt, a bedside ultrasound can be performed to confirm presenting part.

Routine laboratory testing for the laboring woman includes hemoglobin or hematocrit, urinalysis particularly for the hypertensive or diabetic patient, and a tube of blood that can be used for type and crossmatch if blood products are needed emergently. If the woman has had no prenatal care, then a type and antibody screen should be performed as well as infectious disease testing, including human immunodeficiency virus, syphilis, and hepatitis B. (If the woman has received prenatal care, then the results of these tests should be available in the prenatal record.) Some states now require infectious disease testing for all women presenting in labor because a positive result can prompt altered labor management to reduce the risk of vertical transmission to the infant.

Group B *Streptococcus* (GBS) vaginal cultures are recommended for every woman between 35 and 37 weeks of gestation. If the woman has a history of a positive GBS vaginal or urine culture in the current pregnancy, a prior GBS-affected infant, or has completed <37 weeks with an unknown culture status, then prophylactic antibiotics for GBS should be administered during labor (6).

According to the American College of Obstetricians and Gynecologists, fetal heart rate assessment for the uncomplicated, normal laboring patient should be performed at a minimum by intermittent auscultation every 30 minutes immediately following a contraction in the first stage of labor and every 15 minutes in the second stage (2). When continuous electronic fetal heart rate monitoring is being performed, the strip should be assessed every 30 minutes in the first stage and every 15 minutes in the second stage. This time interval allows for some movement of the woman in the labor room or on the labor unit if appropriate and desired.

Laboring women should also be educated regarding options for analgesia, and analgesia should be provided at the patient's request assuming no contraindications. Commonly used analgesia includes epidural anesthesia and IV pain medications. To assist with pain control, a pudendal block or local anesthesia can be provided at the time of delivery. Women with epidural analgesia require IV fluids and vital sign assessment at least every 30 minutes (7).

CLINICAL PEARL

Patients may request an epidural at any time during their labor course. Patients do not have to be dilated 3 to 4 cm prior to getting an epidural.

Option 2: Fair Condition

If the patient is term but has risk factors for labor complications, including but not limited to a history of a prior cesarean section or prior delivery complication, preterm gestation, medical complications of pregnancy, chronic medical illness, or known fetal abnormalities, then the patient and fetus should be followed more closely. Laboratory testing in addition to the previously described routine testing may be indicated, including a complete blood count with platelets, liver function tests, creatinine for hypertensive women, and glucose monitoring for diabetic patients. Continuous IV fluids should be provided and oral intake should be avoided. Anesthesiology should be notified of the admission and may perform an assessment of the patient, as the likelihood of operative intervention and need for anesthesia is higher in this group of patients.

Option 3: Critical Condition

Occasionally, a woman will present with acute issues that require immediate intervention. These include complications such as severe pre-eclampsia, eclampsia, actively bleeding placenta previa, suspected placental abruption, and/or nonreassuring fetal heart tones. In many of these situations, the need for cesarean delivery is likely unless delivery is imminent at presentation.

The patient should not receive anything by mouth, and two large-bore IV accesses should be obtained. The patient should consent to cesarean delivery, and the anesthesiology team must see the patient. Blood products should be crossmatched and available if the patient is bleeding.

The First Few Hours

After you have confirmed that your patient is in active labor, the next few hours are used to determine if she will spontaneously go into labor or if you will need to intervene and augment the process.

History

After admission, the patient should continue to have strong, regular contractions. It is important to continuously assess for any loss of fluid that indicates the rupture of membranes or heavy bleeding. Changes in pain or the sensation of increased pressure in the pelvis may indicate significant progress in labor. Analgesia should be provided to maintain adequate pain control while minimizing any potential side effects (such as hypotension after epidurals).

Physical Examination

Vitals signs should be obtained and fetal monitoring performed as required, based on the protocol of the unit as previously noted. Although not required, serial cervical examination every 1 to 2 hours documenting dilation, effacement, and station during the active phase is sufficient to determine if appropriate progression of labor has occurred (1). Hourly evaluation and examination are indicated in the second stage of labor. If protraction or arrest disorders are suspected based on inadequate progress per the criteria for labor abnormalities noted in Table 2-2, then additional assessment of the contraction strength and frequency is needed, including possible placement of an IUPC.

Labs and Tests to Consider

For the normal laboring patient, no further labs should be needed. For patients with laboratory abnormalities at admission, repeat testing may be appropriate.

Treatment

For the laboring woman making appropriate progress with no signs or symptoms of maternal or fetal morbidity, spontaneous vaginal delivery should be anticipated and preparations made. For labor complicated by fetal heart rate abnormalities or dystocias, additional treatments are indicated, as discussed below.

Fetal Heart Rate Abnormalities

Nothing is responsible for as much angst and stress among obstetricians as potentially concerning findings on a fetal heart tracing. The major reason for this angst is the wide degree of interobserver and intraobserver variability in interpreting these findings. Ironically, there is a high false-positive rate associated with abnormal findings. According to consensus at the National Institute of Child Health and Human Development Research Planning Workshop in 1997, recurrent late or variable decelerations with zero variability and substantial bradycardia with zero variability are patterns that should be considered severely abnormal (8). Short of these findings, however, there is no consensus about what constitutes abnormal fetal heart tracing patterns that are universally worthy of intervention.

Despite these limitations, changes in fetal heart tracing that may indicate changing fetal status should be documented and addressed by the provider as follows (2):

- Uterotonic agents should be discontinued.
- The patient should be positioned in the lateral recumbent position to maximize blood return through the vena cava.
- Oxygen should be given.
- Blood pressure should be measured, as hypotension is a common cause of acute fetal heart rate changes.
- A cervical exam should be done, which serves several purposes:
  - Rapid cervical change or descent may result in fetal decelerations, and delivery may be imminent.
  - Cord prolapse should be excluded as a cause for acute decelerations.
  - The fetal scalp can be stimulated during an exam, and if the fetus has accelerations in response to this stimulus, this is reassuring that the fetus is not hypoxemic.
- Anesthesiology should be notified and preparations for operative delivery made. This includes verifying informed consent for cesarean section or operative vaginal delivery if appropriate and if time allows.
- The patient should be transitioned to operative delivery if the fetal heart tracing remains nonreassuring despite resuscitative efforts.

Labor Dystocias

If labor is not progressing appropriately, the first step is to repeat and/or document the assessment of the three Ps: power, passenger, and pelvis. Placement of an IUPC may be helpful to assess the strength of contractions in women for whom the assessment of contractions by other means is difficult. You should consider the possibility of fetal macrosomia or malposition as a source for protracted labor. Augmentation of labor with oxytocin is indicated if it is determined that the strength or the frequency of contractions is inadequate, or if no clear cause is identified. Amniotomy may shorten the course of labor and reduce the need for oxytocin, but may increase the risk for fever.[9] Cesarean section should be reserved for patients with prolonged arrest disorders, as even women with protracted labors often go on to have vaginal deliveries. Allowing up to 4 hours of adequate contractions or up to 6 hours of augmentation is reasonable prior to proceeding with cesarean section for arrest (3). Operative vaginal delivery may be an option for patients who are completely dilated with protraction or arrest of descent at +2 station or below. The patient also must be apprised of these risks prior to the procedure.

Delivery Preparations

Vaginal Delivery. In anticipation of vaginal delivery, a sterile field should be prepared, including gowns and gloves, towels, sponges or gauze pads, and instruments. The usual instrument set will include a needle driver for perineal repairs; scissors for cutting the cord, for suture, and for the possibility of episiotomy; cord clamp; and hemostats. Lidocaine and syringes for analgesia should be available. The woman is generally placed in the lithotomy position and draped, although alternative birthing positions are equally appropriate in the stable patient. You should wash your hands and sterilely gown and glove for the procedure. The woman should continue to provide expulsive efforts. Massage of the perineum is not recommended at this point because it may increase perineal edema. As the fetal head begins to "crown" (i.e., the labia are parted with expulsive efforts), the provider's hand can be placed at the occiput to guide the head and prevent rapid extension, which could lead to periurethral laceration. Many providers also place a towel in the opposite hand, which is held over the perineum and rectum. In some cases, an episiotomy, which is an incision in the perineal body, may be indicated to allow for delivery. Recent literature does not support the routine use of episiotomy as it increases the risk of third- and fourth-degree perineal lacerations. After the head is fully delivered, you should check for nuchal cords and reduce as appropriate. Rotate the fetal head to a transverse orientation and apply gentle downward traction on the head to aid in delivery of the anterior shoulder. If this does not occur easily, shoulder dystocia may be present. After delivery of the anterior shoulder, the remainder of the delivery should occur spontaneously with expulsive efforts.

Operative vaginal delivery with forceps or a vacuum should be reserved for situations in which it is indicated for diagnosed protraction or the arrest of descent, or for a nonreassuring fetal status during the second stage of labor. Prior to placement of the forceps or vacuum, informed consent should be obtained by the provider, with the indication, risks, and benefits reviewed, including the need for a cesarean in the case of an unsuccessful attempt. Appropriate anesthesia should be administered such that the placement of the device is not compromised by patient discomfort. The position and station of the head is confirmed by digital exam prior to application. Steady traction is applied with expulsive efforts until delivery of the head, at which point the instrument is removed and the remainder of the delivery is completed as previously noted.

Delivery of the placenta should occur within 30 minutes of delivery of the infant. Signs of placental separation include cord lengthening, bleeding, and involution of the uterus. At this point, traction can be applied to the cord to facilitate delivery. A hand can be used to provide upward pressure above the pubic symphysis to ensure that the uterus is not inverted with delivery of the placenta. After delivery of the placenta, it should be inspected to confirm that it is intact. If there is a suspicion that cotyledons may be retained, or if excessive bleeding is encountered, then a manual inspection of the uterine cavity should be performed to evacuate retained products. If the placenta fails to deliver after 30 minutes, a manual extraction of the placenta may be done.

After the placenta delivers, intravenous or intramuscular oxytocin should be given to augment uterine tone as it has been shown to decrease the rate of postpartum hemorrhage. The uterine fundus should also be palpably firm at or below the level of the umbilicus. You should thoroughly examine the cervix, vagina, and perineum, looking for lacerations or signs of trauma. All lacerations should be repaired in a systematic fashion. At the conclusion of the repair, a rectal exam needs to be done to detect occult lacerations or any suture inadvertently entering the rectal mucosa, as these findings would increase the rate of postpartum fistula formation.

Cesarean Section. Once the decision has been made that cesarean delivery is necessary, the patient should be prepared for the operating room. Standard procedures include obtaining consent for the procedure, placement of a Foley catheter, ensuring adequate IV access, and starting continuous IV fluids. Anesthesiology personnel should be present to prepare the patient for anesthesia. If the patient has an epidural catheter in place, additional medication can be given via this route to obtain surgical anesthesia. In non-emergent circumstances, epidural or spinal anesthesia is used most frequently for cesarean delivery because they reduce the risk of maternal aspiration, produce minimal postoperative side effects, and do not sedate the neonate. General anesthesia is reserved for emergent situations when time does not allow for placement of a spinal block, for patients with contraindications to regional anesthesia, or for patients in whom placement of a spinal block is not technically successful. Be aware that spinal and epidural anesthesia can produce profound hypotension via systemic vasodilation, so patients must have adequate hydration prior to placement as well as close monitoring of vital signs with the ability to treat hypotension after placement of regional anesthesia.

Once the aforementioned measures are in place, the patient is prepared and draped for surgery, and the adequacy of analgesia is confirmed. Cesarean sections can be performed through a transverse skin incision (Pfannenstiel) or midline vertical incision, with the former being preferred and more cosmetic. When a patient is full term, the uterus is typically entered via a transverse incision in the developed lower uterine segment. In rare cases, other incisions in the uterus are required, such as the vertical midline, "classic" incision. This type of incision results in more blood loss because it passes through the muscular contractile portion of the uterus and produces scarring that can increase the likelihood of uterine rupture in subsequent pregnancies.

EXTENDED IN-HOSPITAL MANAGEMENT

Following vaginal or cesarean delivery, a period of close observation is necessary, including the assessment of vital signs every 15 to 30 minutes, and serial fundal exams to ensure that uterine tone is adequate and that no heavy bleeding is occurring. Women should be encouraged to initiate breast-feeding as soon as possible following delivery. Approximately 2 hours after delivery in most hospitals, the patient can be transferred to routine postpartum and/or postsurgical care. The standard length of stay is 2 days postpartum for vaginal delivery and 3 days for cesarean delivery, although this may vary depending on the patient's desires and the institutional practice.

DISPOSITION

Discharge Goals

Discharge from the hospital is determined by multiple factors:

- Vital signs demonstrate that the patient is hemodynamically stable.
- Vaginal bleeding is consistent with normal lochia (i.e., moderate to heavy menses), and should continue to improve on a daily basis. Patients should be cautioned that bleeding might temporarily increase with breastfeeding.
- Breast-feeding has been established, and appropriate infant care is demonstrated by the mother.
- The patient has resumed a normal diet, has appropriate bowel and bladder function, and can ambulate and care for herself and her infant at home.
- The patient has appropriate pain control with oral pain medications.

Outpatient Care

The woman should be counseled on the normal postpartum course, including issues related to lactation, mood changes or "baby blues," normal lochia, and pain management. Contraceptive issues should be addressed. The patient should be encouraged to contact the clinic if her symptoms are concerning to her or seem to be outside of the normal expected course. An outpatient visit 4 to 6 weeks following delivery should be arranged, at which point a physical exam, including speculum and bimanual exam, is performed to ascertain normal uterine involution.

WHAT YOU NEED TO REMEMBER

- Active labor is diagnosed when the patient is having regular, painful contractions and cervical change, and the cervix is 3 to 5 cm dilated. At this point, admission to labor and delivery is indicated.
- Although labor is a natural and normal process, intervention may be necessary.
- If fetal heart rate abnormalities exist, a systematic approach to resuscitating the fetus may correct the situation. If the fetal heart tracing is nonreassuring, then the patient should be transitioned to cesarean section or operative vaginal delivery.
- In cases of labor dystocia, an assessment of the cause of the problem and a conservative approach to treatment should be used. If this fails, then cesarean section may be indicated.

REFERENCES

1. Cunningham FG, Leveno KL, Bloom SL, et al. *Williams Obstetrics*. 22nd ed. New York, NY: McGraw-Hill; 2005.
2. American College of Obstetricians and Gynecologists. ACOG practice bulletin number 70, December 2005: Intrapartum fetal heart rate monitoring. *Obstet Gynecol*. 2005;106(6):1453–1460.
3. American College of Obstetricians and Gynecologists. ACOG practice bulletin number 49, December 2003: Dystocia and augmentation of labor. *Obstet Gynecol*. 2003;102:1445–1454.
4. Notson FC, Cnattingius S, Bergsjo P, et al. Cesarean section delivery in the 1980s: international comparison by indication. *Am J Obstet Gynecol*. 1994;170:495–504.
5. American College of Obstetricians and Gynecologists. Practice Bulletin No. 17, June 2000: Operative vaginal delivery. Washington, DC: Author; 2000.
6. American College of Obstetricians and Gynecologists. ACOG committee opinion number 279, December 2002: Prevention of early-onset group B streptococcal disease in newborns. *Obstet Gynecol*. 2002;100:1405–1412.
7. American College of Obstetricians and Gynecologists. ACOG practice bulletin number 36, July 2002: Obstetric analgesia and anesthesia. *Obstet Gynecol*. 2002; 100:177–191.
8. Macones GA, Hankins GD, Spong CY, et al. The 2008 National Institute of Child Health and Human Development Workshop Report on Electronic Fetal Monitoring Update on Definitions, Interpretation, and Research Guidelines. *Obstet Gynecol*. 2008;112:661–666.
9. Smyth RMD, Alldred SK, Markham C. Amniotomy for shortening spontaneous labour. *Cochrane Database Syst Rev*. 2007;4:CD006167. DOI: 10.1002/14651858. CD006167.pub2.

Gestational Diabetes

THE PATIENT ENCOUNTER

A 32-year-old pregnant woman (G3P2) at 27 weeks of gestation presents to the emergency department complaining of fatigue, frequent urination, and increased thirst. She denies any history of medical problems. The patient had prenatal care early in her pregnancy with no complications, but lost her insurance 8 weeks ago and hasn't seen a doctor since. Her capillary blood glucose level is 259 and urinalysis reveals glucosuria. A review of her prenatal chart reveals a normal random glucose level drawn at 10 weeks of gestation.

OVERVIEW

Definition

Gestational diabetes (GDM) is glucose intolerance that begins or is first recognized in pregnancy. The majority of glucose intolerance develops during pregnancy, but a patient may have overt diabetes that was previously unrecognized.

Pathophysiology

Placental production of hormones causes increased insulin resistance and the decreased peripheral uptake of glucose. Human placental lactogen is responsible for the majority of these changes, but other hormones, such as cortisol, growth hormone, and progesterone, may play a role as well.

Epidemiology

The prevalence of GDM varies based on ethnicity and the diagnostic criteria used. The reported prevalence in the United States ranges from 1% to 14%, but is most commonly reported as 2% to 5% (1).

Etiology

There are a number of risk factors that may lead to the development of GDM. They include (1):

- Personal history of abnormal glucose tolerance
- Family history of diabetes
- Age >25 years

TABLE 3-1
White Classification of Pregestational Diabetes

Class	Age of Onset (years)	Duration (years)	Vascular Disease
B	>20	<10	None
C	10–19	10–19	None
D	<10	>20	Benign retinopathy
F	Any	Any	Diabetic nephropathy
R	Any	Any	Proliferative retinopathy
H	Any	Any	Ischemic heart disease
T	Any	Any	Renal transplant

- Hispanic, African, Native American, South Asian, East Asian, or Pacific Island ethnicity
- Body mass index >25
- Previous delivery of infant weighing >9 pounds
- Prior poor obstetric outcome

Classification
Diabetes in pregnancy is classified using the White classification (Table 3-1). An A1 diabetic has GDM that is diet-controlled. An A2 diabetic has GDM that requires insulin. Classes B through T are used for patients with known prepregnancy diabetes.

ACUTE MANAGEMENT AND WORKUP

Most patients with GDM are diagnosed and managed as outpatients; however, you must be aware of the potential complications of GDM and know how to manage severe hyperglycemia.

The First 15 Minutes
The first step in evaluating a patient with severe hyperglycemia is to rule out diabetic ketoacidosis (DKA).

Initial Assessment
A diagnosis of DKA is made in the presence of hyperglycemia, anion gap metabolic acidosis, and ketonemia. A measure of arterial blood gas is used to

determine the degree of acidosis, and bicarbonate should be administered if severe acidemia is present.

Admission Criteria and Level of Care Criteria

DKA is rare in gestational diabetics, but when it does occur, it poses a significant risk to both the mother and fetus. You should closely follow glucose levels, urine ketones, and serum electrolytes. Treatment consists of insulin, aggressive intravenous hydration, and electrolyte repletion.

The First Few Hours

In all pregnant patients, it is important to check and monitor the status of the fetus. This can be done by checking intermittent fetal heart tones with a Doppler study. More extended fetal monitoring may be indicated in certain patients, such as those with DKA. In patients with DKA, it is also important to remember that evidence of fetal compromise usually resolves once the mother's academia is corrected.

History

Queries of risk assessment are useful in the counseling related to the risk of developing GDM with subsequent pregnancies. Nevertheless, a family history of diabetes, a prior unexplained stillbirth, or a history of large babies may raise your index of suspicion toward undiagnosed glucose intolerance. In patients with a known history of insulin-dependent diabetes, the patient's age and the duration of the disease are important elements of GDM classification.

CLINICAL PEARL

History alone is not accurate—nearly a third of women afflicted with GDM have no identifiable risk factors.

Physical Examination

In addition to assessments of fetal well-being, your patient should be thoroughly evaluated for evidence of end-organ dysfunction secondary to diabetes. Patients should have a baseline eye exam to look for proliferative retinopathy. A careful cardiac exam should be performed with attention given to blood pressure and identification of an unknown ischemic event.

Labs and Tests to Consider

Key labs and tests to consider include the following:

- Hemoglobin A1c
- 24-hour urine collections for quantitative protein and creatinine (helps establish a baseline if faced with gestational hypertension later in pregnancy)

- Serum creatinine
- 1- and 3-hour glucose tolerance test (GTT; see "Screening" section)
- Anatomic survey at 18 to 21 weeks of gestation for structural fetal anomalies

Treatment

The key to the treatment of GDM is glucose control. Gestational diabetes is managed with either diet or insulin. After a diagnosis of GDM is made, the patient should be initiated on a 1- to 2-week trial of an American Diabetes Association diet. If the patient is unable to maintain fasting blood sugar levels below 105 mg/dL, maintain 2-hour fasting blood sugar levels below 120 mg/dL, or both, pharmacologic therapy should be initiated (2). Insulin is the traditional and most commonly used pharmacologic agent for the treatment of GDM; however, more recent evidence supports the use of glyburide during pregnancy (3). The American College of Obstetricians and Gynecologists does not endorse the use of oral antihyperglycemic agents during pregnancy (2).

CLINICAL PEARL

The goals for blood sugar control in all gestational diabetic women regardless of therapy is a fasting blood sugar level <105 mg/dL and 2-hour fasting blood sugar levels below 120 mg/dL.

EXTENDED INHOSPITAL MANAGEMENT

The goal of inpatient management, if needed, is to obtain optimal glycemic control. It also provides you with an excellent opportunity to ensure that the patient receives diabetic teaching. While admitted, these patients should be seen by a dietician and be counseled regarding American Diabetes Association diet recommendations. They should also be taught how to check their own blood glucose levels and record them in a log. All insulin-requiring diabetics should be taught how to inject insulin.

DISPOSITION

Discharge Goals

Discharge from the hospital is determined by multiple factors. Effective blood sugar control is just one of the few components necessary prior to the release of a patient from direct inhospital supervision. A clear understanding of the blood sugar goals and treatment plan is essential. An appreciation for the management of hyperglycemia and hypoglycemia is necessary for both the patient and her extended support group.

Outpatient Care

After an intensive inpatient program of education and pharmacologic therapy, serial assessment of compliance is important. Fasting blood sugar levels along with monitoring of the daily blood sugar log helps in ascertaining the level of compliance and adequacy of drug dosing. If you are concerned about the accuracy of the reported data, one strategy is to look at the actual glucometer and view the historical log.

Screening

Options for GDM screening include universal screening or selective screening based on risk factors. The recommendation from the 1997 International Workshop on GDM is screening of all women unless they are deemed to be low risk. Low-risk women are those that are members of an ethnic group with a low prevalence of GDM, no known diabetes in a first-degree relative, age younger than 25 years old, normal prepregnancy weight, no history of abnormal glucose metabolism, and no history of poor obstetric outcome (4). Women with a high risk of GDM should have blood glucose testing performed early in the pregnancy. If GDM is not diagnosed at that time, the screening should be repeated at 24 to 28 weeks. All other women should be screened at 24 to 28 weeks (Table 3-2).

Screening for GDM is performed using a 1-hour, 50-g GTT. Different threshold glucose levels for the 1-hour GTT may be used depending on the desired sensitivity. Use of a threshold value of >140 mg/dL will detect approximately 80% of women with GDM, while use of a lower cutoff value of >130 mg/dL will increase sensitivity to approximately 90%. If the 1-hour GTT is elevated, a diagnostic 3-hour GTT with a 100-g load is performed.

TABLE 3-2
Diagnostic Criteria for Gestational Diabetes Mellitus

Status	Plasma or Serum Glucose Level Carpenter/Coustan Conversion		Plasma Level National Diabetes Data Group Conversion	
	(mg/dL)	(mmol/L)	(mg/dL)	(mmol/L)
Fasting	95	5.3	105	5.8
1 hour	180	10.0	190	10.6
2 hours	155	8.6	165	9.2
3 hours	140	7.8	145	8.0

The 100-g GTT is administered with the patient fasting. Serum glucose levels are obtained in the fasting state, along with levels at 1, 2, and 3 hours after the 100-g load. The test is considered positive if two or more thresholds are met or exceeded. There are two diagnostic criteria commonly used, as listed in Table 3-2.

Women with a random glucose level >200 mg/dL or a fasting glucose level >126 mg/dL do not need to be screened. These values, if confirmed, are diagnostic of diabetes and these women should be treated as gestational diabetics (4).

Counseling

GDM is associated with an increased risk of both fetal and maternal morbidity. Patients with GDM have an increased risk of pre-eclampsia, fetal macrosomia, cesarean delivery, and birth trauma. There is also a higher incidence of perinatal mortality and the infant is at risk for neonatal complications, including hyperbilirubinemia, hypoglycemia, and hypocalcemia. Additionally, women with GDM have an increased risk of developing diabetes later in life. Therefore, all women with GDM should be evaluated for hyperglycemia at 6 to 12 weeks postpartum. Screening for diabetes mellitus should be repeated at a minimum of 3-year intervals (4). A recent systematic review reported that the cumulative incidence of the future development of diabetes ranged from 2.6 to 70%, with the greatest increase in risk occurring during the first 5 years after pregnancy (5).

WHAT YOU NEED TO REMEMBER

- GDM is glucose intolerance that begins or is first recognized in pregnancy.
- Human placental lactogen is the primary hormone responsible for GDM.
- All pregnant women should be screened unless they are deemed to be low risk.
- Screening for GDM is performed using a 1-hour GTT. If this is elevated, a diagnostic 3-hour GTT should be performed. A diagnosis of GDM is made if two or more values are elevated.
- Treatment consists of glucose control. Dietary therapy is attempted first; however, if glucose levels remain elevated, insulin is initiated.
- In the White classification, an A1 diabetic has GDM that is diet-controlled. An A2 diabetic has GDM that requires insulin.
- GDM is associated with an increased risk of both fetal and maternal morbidity.
- Women with GDM have an increased risk of developing diabetes later in life.

REFERENCES

1. American College of Obstetrics and Gynecology. ACOG practice bulletin number 30, September 2001: Gestational diabetes. *Obstet Gynecol.* 2001;98:525–538.
2. Cunningham FG, Leveno KJ, Bloom SL, et al. *Williams Obstetrics.* 22nd ed. New York, NY: McGraw-Hill; 2005:1175.
3. Coustan DR. Pharmacological management of gestational diabetes. *Diabetes Care.* 2007;39:S208–S208.
4. American Diabetes Association. Position statement: gestational diabetes Mellitus. *Diabetes Care.* 2004;27: S88–S90.
5. Kim C, Newton KM, Knopp RH. Gestational diabetes and the incidence of type 2 diabetes. *Diabetes Care.* 2002;25(10):1862–1868.

Shoulder Dystocia

THE PATIENT ENCOUNTER

You are called to Room 4 on the labor and delivery suite by the nurse to attend the delivery of a 25-year-old pregnant woman (G2P1001). Her first delivery was an uncomplicated vaginal delivery of a healthy male infant who weighed 6 pounds and 4 ounces. This pregnancy has been uncomplicated and she presented to labor and delivery in active labor about 6 hours ago. Her labor has progressed well with augmentation using a low dose of pitocin. You have the patient push and deliver the head without problems. You then have her push to deliver the anterior shoulder; however, the infant doesn't budge and the shoulder seems to be stuck behind the pubic symphysis.

OVERVIEW

Definition

The case described here deals with the clinical picture of shoulder dystocia. This is perhaps one of the scariest scenarios that the obstetrician may encounter on the labor and delivery ward. However, it is a situation that the obstetrician should be prepared for at every delivery. Shoulder dystocia is described as delivery of the fetal head but prevention of further expulsion of the infant by the impaction of the fetal shoulders within the maternal pelvis. This chapter will deal with the risk factors for shoulder dystocia that should alert the physician to an increased risk for a difficult delivery, as well as the various maneuvers that are employed to help relieve the dystocia and deliver the infant.

Pathophysiology

Disproportion between the maternal pelvis and the presenting fetal shoulder is one of the main factors responsible for a shoulder dystocia. The issue can be primarily maternal or fetal in origin. Maternal factors include pelvic irregularity from trauma or small maternal habitus. Fetal factors can include congenital anomalies, tumors, and even male gender of the fetus.

Epidemiology

Most sources quote an incidence for shoulder dystocia to be between 0.6% and 1.7%. The difference in the incidence in these studies is most likely a result of differences in the populations studied. Some studies even show an increase in the incidence over time, which is likely the result of increasing birth weights and increased documentation of dystocia.

Etiology

Although it is true that many cases of shoulder dystocia are completely random and unpredictable, there are some risk factors that have been identified that should alert the physician to the increased risk of encountering a shoulder dystocia. Maternal risk factors include maternal obesity, multiparity, and diabetes. All these probably exert their influences because of effects on fetal birth weight. Many studies have shown a relationship between increasing birth weight and an increased incidence of shoulder dystocia. Rouse and Owen (1) determined that 1,000 cesarean deliveries would have to be performed on macrosomic newborns to prevent one permanent brachial plexus injury. Hence, the American College of Obstetricians and Gynecologists (2) has recommended that a planned cesarean section may be considered for suspected fetal macrosomia when fetal weight exceeds 4,500 g in a diabetic patient or >5,000 g in a nondiabetic patient. Table 4-1 lists other common antepartum and intrapartum risk factors.

CLINICAL PEARL

You may recommend a planned cesarean section if the estimated fetal weight exceeds 4,500 g in a diabetic patient or exceeds 5,000 g in a nondiabetic patient.

Although these risk factors should alert you to the possibility of the development of a shoulder dystocia, you should also remember that many

TABLE 4-1
Risk Factors for Shoulder Dystocia

Antepartum Risk Factors	Intrapartum Risk Factors
1. Maternal diabetes	1. Prolonged first or second stage of labor
2. Macrosomia	2. Induction of labor
3. Postterm pregnancy	3. Operative vaginal delivery
4. Maternal obesity	
5. History of previous shoulder dystocia	
6. History of prior macrosomic infant	

cases of shoulder dystocia cannot be accurately predicted. You should always be prepared to deal in a timely fashion with the development of shoulder dystocia.

ACUTE MANAGEMENT AND WORKUP

When a shoulder dystocia is encountered, the delivery room quickly becomes a very chaotic place. The most important thing to remember is to remain calm.

The First 15 Minutes

The first step is to quickly assess the situation and bring together whatever people or equipment may be needed.

Initial Assessment

The job of the delivering physician is to help effect a quick and safe delivery of the infant and the only way to do this is by remaining calm and in control.

1. Have someone mark the time that the dystocia is encountered. This will help when documenting the incident as well as give you an accurate idea of how long you have been attempting delivery of the infant.
2. Call for help. If available, have other residents brought in as well as extra nurses.
3. Have a pediatrician called to help with resuscitation of the infant if needed.
4. Have someone check to make sure that an operating room is open and available if needed.

Physical Examination

Shoulder dystocia is a clinical diagnosis. There are no tests or images that need to be obtained to prove the diagnosis. The initial physical examination is geared toward helping the obstetrician assess the order of resuscitative maneuvers. Identifying the presenting shoulder and the position of the head will help with guiding the direction of rotation and/or pressure.

Treatment

When dystocia is encountered, the physician must act quickly to deliver the infant as soon as possible. Over the years, multiple maneuvers have been developed that are thought to help effect delivery of the infant. No one maneuver has been found to be superior to any other, and the order of execution is based on your preference. When a shoulder dystocia is encountered, most clinicians go through the maneuvers one after another until the infant is successfully delivered.

McRoberts Maneuver

The McRoberts maneuver is often quoted as the most successful technique to resolve a shoulder dystocia. It involves having assistants help place the patient's legs in an exaggerated flexion position (Fig. 4-1). This helps to straighten out the sacrum with regard to the lumbar spine and rotates the pubic symphysis toward the maternal head. This then allows for the impacted shoulder to free itself and the infant may then be delivered. In some laboratory models, it has been shown that the McRoberts maneuver decreases the incidence of both fetal clavicular fracture and brachial plexus injury.

Suprapubic Pressure

Suprapubic pressure involves having an assistant apply pressure above the pubic symphysis at a 45-degree angle from the vertical in order to try and move the fetal shoulder down and toward the fetal chest so that the infant can pass under the symphysis. The important point here is to make sure that the assistant is applying force above the symphysis and not directly on it or on the uterine fundus.

Rubin Maneuver

The Rubin maneuver is used to try to decrease the shoulder circumference and transverse diameter by abducting the most accessible shoulder, which is

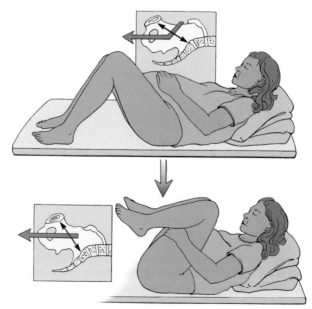

FIGURE 4-1: Shoulder dystocia technique: the McRoberts maneuver.

typically the anterior shoulder. The operator's fingers are used to place pressure on the back of the shoulder, pushing it toward the fetal chest. Essentially, this makes the shoulder circumference smaller and allows for the infant to slip beneath the symphysis.

Wood Maneuver

The Wood maneuver is also referred to as the *screw maneuver*. It is based on the notion that the fetus acts like a screw as it passes through the birth canal. The fetal shoulders can be thought of as passing through a threaded passage formed by the pubic symphysis, the sacral promontory, and the coccyx. If thought of in this way, then it would make sense that a direct pulling force would not be the best way to deliver the infant. The Wood maneuver tries to dislodge the infant by causing the fetal shoulders to make a spiral motion as the infant is delivered. In this maneuver, the left hand of the operator is used to make a downward thrust on the infant's buttocks transabdominally, while at the same time two fingers from the right hand are used to place pressure on the posterior aspect of the posterior shoulder and the shoulder is gently rotated in a clockwise direction (Fig. 4-2). This causes the infant to act like a screw and spiral as it is delivered.

Posterior Arm Extraction

This maneuver is accomplished by delivering the posterior arm first, which should decrease the fetal shoulder circumference and then allow the infant to slip beneath the symphysis. The hand you use is determined by which way the fetal back lies. If the fetal back is lying toward the maternal left, then you use your left hand. If the back lies toward the maternal right, then you use your right hand. You slide your hand along the curvature of the maternal sacrum, allowing it to slide down the fetal humorous to the level of the antecubital fossa. Pressure is then applied at this area to cause the fetal arm to flex. At this point, the fetal forearm is grasped and swept across the fetal chest and face until it is delivered out of the vagina. This should then allow more room posteriorly so that the anterior shoulder is dislodged and the infant is delivered.

CLINICAL PEARL

No one maneuver has been found to be superior to any other, and the order of execution is based on your preference. When a shoulder dystocia is encountered, most clinicians go through the maneuvers one after another until the infant is successfully delivered.

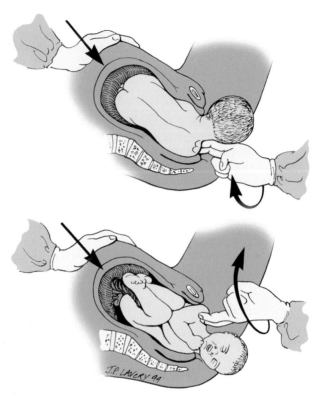

FIGURE 4-2: Shoulder dystocia technique: the Wood corkscrew maneuver.

Heroic Measures

There are times when the fetus in unable to be delivered despite the appropriate use of the maneuvers mentioned previously. In that rare instance, the maneuvers are repeated or further actions may be considered. The following measures have been described to help deliver an infant when all other measures have failed. It should be noted that these measures are to be used as a last resort and are associated with a much higher incidence of fetal morbidity and mortality.

Intentional Clavicle Fracture

This maneuver reduces the diameter of the fetal shoulders by breaking one of the fetal clavicles. The bone is broken by using the operator's fingers to place pressure on the clavicle at the midportion of the bone and press upwards toward the fetal head. This will hopefully cause the bone to break outward, away from the subclavian vessels and pleural space.

Abdominal Rescue

This maneuver involves performing a low transverse hysterotomy and using the operator's hands to manually pass the fetal shoulders below the pubic symphysis. The fetus may then be delivered vaginally.

Zavanelli Maneuver

This is another maneuver that has been developed for use when all other options have been exhausted and the fetus is still undelivered. It involves using subcutaneous terbutaline to relax the uterus, followed by manual replacement of the fetal head into the intravaginal location. The fetus is then delivered by emergency cesarean section.

EXTENDED IN-HOSPITAL MANAGEMENT

Shoulder dystocia carries with it the danger of complications for both the fetus and mother. Following delivery of the fetus, it should be passed off to the waiting pediatrician so that it can be quickly evaluated and treated as necessary. Meanwhile, the mother should be evaluated for any further treatment that she may need.

Maternal complications include both physical and psychological. The physical complications include postpartum hemorrhage from both atony and lower genital tract lacerations that may be accidentally created during the difficult delivery. Uterotonic agents may be used to treat the atonic uterus, and any bleeding lacerations should be repaired. Another possible complication includes a transient femoral neuropathy that may appear following the use of the McRoberts maneuver. This neuropathy is generally short-lived and does not require any specific treatment. The damage caused by shoulder dystocia also includes a psychological element in the mother. The delivery room during a shoulder dystocia is typically a loud and chaotic place. Time should be taken at the end of the delivery to adequately explain exactly what happened and what measures were taken to help deliver the fetus. This conversation should be summarized in the delivery note.

Fetal complications of shoulder dystocia include brachial plexus injuries, bone fractures, and the complications of fetal asphyxia. The incidence of brachial plexus injury following shoulder dystocia ranges from 10% to 20%. These injuries include both Erb-Duchenne and Klumpke palsies, depending on which nerve roots are damaged. Fortunately, most of these infants recover function of the affected arm by 6 months to 1 year. The risk of broken bones is less than that with brachial plexus injury and, when encountered, the clavicle is the most commonly injured bone. The risk of fetal asphyxia increases with the increased time that it takes to deliver the fetus.

DISPOSITION

Discharge Goals

A delayed postpartum hemorrhage and/or endometritis will typically present within the first 36 hours postpartum. After the patient has been deemed stable using the standard postvaginal delivery criteria, the patient is safe to be discharged home. The disposition of the infant rests in the hands of the pediatricians.

Outpatient Care

Outpatient care is no different than that of a typical vaginal delivery. In the case of a transient femoral neuropathy, serial neurologic examinations are appropriate to document continued improvement.

WHAT YOU NEED TO REMEMBER

- Shoulder dystocia is an obstetrical emergency, and the goal of treatment should be the quick and safe delivery of the fetus.
- Although there are multiple risk factors that have been linked to shoulder dystocia, they do not always accurately predict which patient will develop this complication.
- The first step is always to call for help.
- There are multiple maneuvers that have been described to deal with shoulder dystocia. The physician should be well versed in the use of these maneuvers.
- Following the delivery of the fetus, time should be taken to explain to the patient what happened during the delivery, and all of her questions should be adequately answered. The delivery note should be specific as to what maneuvers were used during delivery and should include a summary of the conversation with the patient at the end of the delivery.

REFERENCES

1. Rouse DJ, Owen J. Prophylactic cesarean delivery for fetal macrosomia diagnosed by means of ultrasonography: a Faustian bargain? *Am J Obstet Gynecol.* 1999;181: 332–338.
2. American College of Obstetricians and Gynecologists. ACOG practice bulletin number 40, 2002. Shoulder dystocia. *Obstet Gynecol.* 2002;100:1045–1050.

SUGGESTED READINGS

Cunningham FG, Leveno KJ, Bloom SL, et al. *Williams Obstetrics.* 22nd ed. New York, NY: McGraw-Hill; 2005.

Gabbe SG, Niebyl JR, Simpson JL. *Obstetrics: Normal and Problem Pregnancies.* 4rth ed. New York, NY: Churchill Livingstone; 2002:493–498.

Gilstrap LC, Cunningham FG, Vandorsten JP. Dystocia: Abnormal labor. In: *Operative Obstetrics.* 2nd ed. New York, NY: McGraw-Hill; 2002:199–221.

Pre-Eclampsia, Eclampsia, and HELLP Syndrome

THE PATIENT ENCOUNTER

A healthy, 17-year-old African American woman (G1P0) calls your nurse at 39 weeks of gestation complaining of a severe headache and "seeing spots." Her baseline blood pressure at 16 weeks of gestation was 108/62 mm Hg. The nurse urges her to come to triage and you are then notified of her vital signs. On arrival, her blood pressure is 162/118 mm Hg and her heart rate is 98 beats per minute. Her weight is 161 pounds and she complains of swelling in her hands, feet, and face. Her urine dipstick test reveals no glucose and a protein level of 4+.

OVERVIEW

Definition

Blood pressure in pregnancy usually decreases because of the natural incidence of reduced vascular resistance. Blood pressure is usually lowest during the second trimester and begins to rise again during the third trimester. However, blood pressure should not rise higher than the normal value before pregnancy. High blood pressure in pregnancy can be sorted into different categories depending on the gestational age, the quantity of protein that is measured, and the severity of systolic and diastolic blood pressure. Those who have hypertension prior to pregnancy are classified in the category of chronic hypertension. A blood pressure of 140/90 mm Hg or more measured prior to 20 weeks of gestation is consistent with chronic hypertension.

If pregnancy induces high blood pressure after 20 weeks, it is called *gestational hypertension*. Proteinuria is what separates pre-eclampsia from gestational hypertension. Hypertension with >300 mg of protein in the urine measured over 24 hours is called *pre-eclampsia*. In women with known chronic hypertension, new-onset proteinuria or worsening blood pressures after 24 weeks of gestation help confirm the diagnosis of *pre-eclampsia superimposed on chronic hypertension. Eclampsia* is when a seizure occurs with pre-eclampsia.

Pre-eclampsia is further subdivided into mild pre-eclampsia and severe pre-eclampsia. Mild pre-eclampsia is defined as a systolic blood pressure between 140 and 160 mm Hg, or a diastolic blood pressure between 90 and 110 mm Hg. This must be accompanied with proteinuria >300 mg over

24 hours or a urine dipstick level of 2+ or more. The criteria for severe pre-eclampsia are a systolic blood pressure >160 mm Hg, a diastolic blood pressure >110 mm Hg, >5 g of urine protein in a 24-hour collection, or >3+ protein on a urine dipstick. In addition, severe pre-eclampsia can be associated with hallmark symptoms, such as altered mental state, headache, visual disturbances, and midepigastric or right upper quadrant pain.

Pathophysiology

Complications from untreated pre-eclampsia or eclampsia can, in the worst-case scenarios, lead to maternal death, especially in areas where access to care is limited. The treatment for severe pre-eclampsia or eclampsia, regardless of gestation, is delivery. No definitive cause has been identified yet, but promising research is in development. The underlying pathophysiology is generally accepted to involve changes in the activity of blood vessels. There is alternating arteriolar constriction or vasospasm, which leads to the usual rise and fall of blood pressure and other symptoms, such as headache and visual changes. Intravascular depletion secondary to transudative edema can produce other symptoms. This phenomenon is also known as *vasospasm* and *leaky vessels*. The vasospasm and the endothelial damage are what lead to local tissue hypoxemia. Hypoxemia leads to hemolysis, necrosis, and end-organ damage. Complications of this process can include placental abruption, coagulopathies, renal failure, hepatic rupture, and even fetal death.

Epidemiology

According to the National Center for Health Statistics in 2001, gestational hypertension afflicted approximately 4% of all pregnancies in the United States (1). Nulliparous women and women at both ends of the reproductive age spectrum are most commonly affected.

Etiology

Although the origin of pre-eclampsia is unclear, there are certain risk factors that may help to identify patients who may be at risk. A prior history of pre-eclampsia or a family history of pre-eclampsia is often identified. Other risk factors include nulliparity; African American race; chronic hypertension; extremes of age, such as those women who are younger than 18 or older than 35; diabetes; chronic renal disease; and multiple gestations, such as twins or triplets.

ACUTE MANAGEMENT AND WORKUP

Correct identification of where in the spectrum of hypertensive diseases the patient currently lies is critical to the appropriate management of the mother and fetus.

The First 15 Minutes

Rapid assessment of fetal well-being and maternal stability are the primary goals of the first 15 minutes. This allows the provider time to recruit the resources necessary to deliver the most appropriate care.

Initial Assessment

The initial assessment of any patient should always include a history and physical examination. Important data you should obtain include prior blood pressure readings, a record of weight gain, and prior urinalysis. Laboratory tests should include a complete blood count with platelets, serum creatinine, liver function tests, and a urine dipstick for proteinuria. Table 5-1 provides a summary of the diagnosis criteria.

Admission Criteria and Level of Care Criteria

These patients are typically admitted for in-hospital monitoring of serial blood pressures. Bed rest may be beneficial to those with mild pre-eclampsia. Delivery is indicated for severe pre-eclampsia regardless of the estimated gestational age of the fetus. Severe-range blood pressures should be treated with an intravenous antihypertensive such as hydralazine or labetalol. An anticonvulsant, such as magnesium sulfate, should also be started and continued for 24 hours after the time of delivery.

> **CLINICAL PEARL**
>
> *Severe pre-eclampsia is an indication for immediate delivery regardless of the gestational age of the fetus.*

If the patient has experienced an eclamptic seizure, you should not attempt delivery until the patient is stable. Fetal heart rate decelerations may be seen after a seizure. It is not necessary to perform a cesarean section immediately unless there are maternal or fetal indications that warrant a cesarean section. After delivery, the patient should be monitored closely, including monitoring of vital signs and urine output. It is not uncommon that patients with severe-range blood pressures will continue to require an intravenous antihypertensive after delivery or when fluid shifting occurs.

> **CLINICAL PEARL**
>
> *In the setting of a patient experiencing an eclamptic seizure, treating and stabilizing the mother will ultimately treat any fetal heart rate decelerations. Eclampsia itself is not an indication for an emergent cesarean section.*

TABLE 5-1
Diagnostic Criteria for Hypertensive Disorders in Pregnancy[a]

Chronic HTN	Gestational HTN	Pre-Eclampsia	Eclampsia	HELLP Syndrome
BP >140/90 before 20 wk	BP >140/90 after 20 wk	BP >140/90 after 20 wk (minimum) but usually >160/110	BP >140/90 with seizures	Pre-eclampsia with end-organ damage
Any degree of proteinuria	No proteinuria	Proteinuria >300 mg/ 24 hr	—	Hemolysis, elevated liver enzymes, low platelets
Normal lab values	Normal lab values	AST >90, creatinine >1.0, platelets <100,000	—	May be associated with coagulopathies
No symptoms; headache usually relieved by Tylenol	No symptoms; headache usually relieved by Tylenol	Headache not usually relieved by Tylenol, visual changes, midepigastric or RUQ pain	Seizure activity that can not be explained by other causes	Requires close monitoring

[a]HTN, hypertension; HELLP, hemolysis, elevated liver enzymes, and low platelets; BP, blood pressure; AST, aspartate aminotransferase; RUQ, right upper quadrant.

The level of care, including intensive care unit monitoring, should be decided on an individual case basis. Because delivery is the cure for pre-eclampsia or eclampsia, the signs and symptoms associated with this disease process should improve within a few hours to a few days. Some patients may have more severe complications, such as pulmonary edema, intracranial hemorrhage, temporary occipital lobe blindness, liver hematoma rupture, or other serious damage to other internal organs. Some of these symptoms can be seen with HELLP syndrome, which will be discussed later in the chapter.

The First Few Hours

In the case of severe pre-eclampsia, aggressive antihypertensive and anticonvulsant therapy must be initiated without delay to avoid catastrophic maternal and fetal morbidity.

History

Throughout the labor course, continue to communicate with the patient and monitor her for any signs of neurologic impairment, excessive drowsiness secondary to magnesium toxicity, or new symptoms such as headache or blurry vision. These may be symptoms of an impending seizure. Continue to treat severe-range blood pressures aggressively.

Physical Examination

Perform a complete neurological examination. Check for deep tendon reflexes every hour while the patient is receiving magnesium. Pre-eclampsia will lead to hypertonic reflexes, whereas magnesium toxicity will first manifest with hypotonic reflexes. Monitor the oxygen saturation frequently. A record of intake and output should be strictly monitored. Monitor the patient's weight every day.

Labs and Tests to Consider

All of the labs should be serially evaluated. Any abnormal value should be monitored frequently to ensure resolution of pre-eclampsia or eclampsia. It may be necessary to transfuse a pre-eclamptic patient if she experiences acute blood loss, as these patients typically do not have the usual volume expansion seen in pregnancy. If platelets fall below 20,000, a transfusion of platelets may be necessary.

Imaging

Imaging is usually not necessary except in cases of an eclamptic seizure. Magnetic resonance imaging or computed tomographic scanning of the head is useful in cases of acute neurologic changes or trauma from a fall.

Treatment

Treatment goals include blood pressure management, seizure prevention, and delivery of the infant, in cases of severe pre-eclampsia. A single

TABLE 5-2
Clinical Manifestations Based on Serum Magnesium Sulfate Concentrations

Concentration of Serum Magnesium Sulfate (mg/mL)	Clinical Response
4–7	Therapeutic level
8	CNS depression
12	Loss of deep tendon reflexes
>15	Respiratory depression, heart block, and cardiac arrest

course of corticosteroids should be given to all women between 24 and 34 weeks of gestation who are at risk for preterm delivery within 7 days. Intravenous hydralazine or labetalol to acutely treat severe-range blood pressures in pregnancy are usually first-line therapy. Magnesium sulfate is initiated for seizure prophylaxis. An intravenous loading dose of 4 to 6 g is first administered. A maintenance level is then started at 2 g/h, with serum magnesium levels re-evaluated at 2, 4, and 12 hours to ensure a therapeutic level. A level too low may allow seizure breakthrough. A high level could lead to respiratory depression, coma, or cardiac arrest (Table 5-2).

The magnesium sulfate infusion is continued for 24 hours postpartum. Eclampsia can still develop after completion of infusion of magnesium sulfate. If this occurs, magnesium sulfate should be reinitiated and continued until 24 hours after the onset of convulsions.

EXTENDED INHOSPITAL MANAGEMENT

The HELLP syndrome (Hemolysis, Elevated Liver enzymes, and Low Platelets) can be seen in 6 to 8% of pregnancies that are complicated with hypertensive disease. Possible complications include cardiac dysfunction, pulmonary edema, respiratory failure, liver failure, intracranial hemorrhage, coma, and death. The syndrome usually resolves after delivery, but patients may still continue to decompensate before the symptoms improve. It is often best to monitor these patients in an acute care facility or in the intensive care unit.

DISPOSITION

Discharge Goals

The first 24 to 48 hours postpartum are critical in confirming normalization of the hypertensive disease process. Once your patient begins to mobilize the excess fluid in the form of increased urine output, reductions in blood pressure should follow. In the absence of any further neurologic symptoms, the patient may be discharged home with outpatient monitoring of blood pressure.

Outpatient Care

Depending on the severity of disease, many obstetricians have pre-eclamptic patients return for a blood pressure check approximately 2 weeks after delivery. If the patient's blood pressure is normal, additional lab work is not necessary. If the patient's blood pressure remains elevated, continued surveillance is necessary to exclude an undiagnosed chronic process.

WHAT YOU NEED TO REMEMBER

- If you are managing a patient with high blood pressure, you must decide what category she is in—chronic hypertension, gestational hypertension, or pre-eclampsia.
- Be aware of the gestational age of the fetus.
- Check a urine dipstick, as well as levels of hematocrit, platelets, aspartate aminotransferase, and creatinine.
- Abnormal platelets are <100,000.
- Abnormal aspartate aminotransferase is >90.
- Abnormal creatinine is >1.0.
- Severe range blood pressures are >160 mm Hg systolic and >110 mm Hg diastolic.
- Treat severe-range blood pressures with intravenous hydralazine or labetalol.
- Delivery is the cure.
- Don't panic if the patient has an eclamptic seizure—treat with intravenous magnesium.
- Continue magnesium for 24 hours postpartum.

REFERENCES

1. Martin JA, Hamilton BE, Ventura SS, et al. Births: final data for 2001. National Vital Statistics Report, Vol. 51, No. 2. Hyattsville, MD: National Center for Health Statistics; 2002.

SUGGESTED READINGS

American College of Obstetricians and Gynecologists. ACOG technical bulletin number 33,2002: Diagnosis and management of preeclampsia and eclampsia. *Obstet Gynecol.* 2002;99:159–167.

American College of Obstetricians and Gynecologists. ACOG committee opinion number 402: Antenatal corticosteroid therapy for fetal maturation. *Obstet Gynecol.* 2008;111:805–807.

Cunningham FG, Leveno KJ, Bloom SL, et al. Hypertensive disorders in pregnancy. In: *Williams Obstetrics.* 22nd ed. New York, NY: McGraw-Hill; 2005:761–808.

Davey DA, MacGillivray I. The classification and definition of the hypertensive disorders of pregnancy. *Am J Obstet Gynecol.* 1988;158:892–898.

Martin JN Jr, Blake PG, Perry KG Jr, McCaul JF, Hess LW, Martin RW. The natural history of HELLP syndrome: patterns of disease progression and regression. *Am J Obstet Gynecol.* 1991;164:1500–1513.

Weinstein L. Syndrome of hemolysis, elevated liver enzymes and low platelet count: a severe consequence of hypertension in pregnancy. *Am J Obstet Gynecol.* 1982;142:159–167.

6

Preterm Labor

THE PATIENT ENCOUNTER

You are called urgently to see a patient who was sent in by the nurse at her obstetrician's office. She is a 23-year-old woman (G3P1011) at 27 weeks gestational age by last menstrual period. She is contracting every 3 to 5 minutes and has to stop talking and breathe through every third contraction. Fetal heart tones are being monitored and are reactive. The contractions are being traced with tocometry, as noted. A cervical exam has not yet been performed.

OVERVIEW

Definition

Preterm birth is a birth that takes place before 37 completed weeks of gestation. It is important to realize that contractions alone are not preterm labor. Instead, preterm labor is defined as regular, painful uterine contractions with cervical dilation and/or effacement.

Pathophysiology

The processes thought to result in preterm labor are mostly unknown. Nevertheless, a few hypothesized mechanisms of preterm delivery have been suggested, such as the activation of the maternal or fetal hypothalamic-pituitary-adrenal (HPA) axis, infection, decidual hemorrhage, and pathologic uterine distention.

Activation of the HPA axis by maternal stress has been associated with a slightly higher rate of preterm delivery, while fetal HPA activation from the stress of uteroplacental vasculopathy has a higher correlation with preterm delivery. The mechanism is thought to consist of an increased release of corticotrophin-releasing hormone, which increases prostaglandin release and can increase myometrial contractility. Additionally, there is an increased release of fetal pituitary adrenocorticotropic hormone, which is thought to stimulate production of placental estrogenic compounds that can stimulate the myometrium.

Inflammation from infection is also postulated to contribute to preterm labor. Ascending genital infections can instigate a systemic inflammatory response and cause preterm labor. Here, the mechanism is thought to result from the cellular release of proinflammatory mediators. Bacteria can also produce an inflammatory response but it is also thought to directly stimulate uterine contractions via endotoxins and other produced products.

Other mechanical sources of preterm labor include vaginal and decidual bleeding. For these, the mechanisms are not clear.

Uterine distension, from processes such as multiple gestations or polyhydramnios, can stretch the myometrium and induce the formation of gap junctions, increase oxytocin receptors, and increase prostaglandin production. These can result in uterine contractions and cervical dilation.

Epidemiology

Preterm labor accounts for 40% to 50% of all preterm births. The difficulty in assessing and treating preterm labor is determining which labors will result in delivery. Conversely, approximately half of all patients hospitalized for preterm labor will deliver at term.

Prevalence and Incidence

As recently as 2006, in the United States, 12.8% of births occurred preterm, and 2% of these were <32 weeks of gestation (1). Half of these preterm births are thought to be a consequence of preterm labor.

Etiology

Although the cause of preterm labor is idiopathic in 30% to 50% of cases, a few sources have been identified. In addition to those discussed in the "Pathophysiology" section, other causes include multiple gestations, preterm prolonged rupture of membranes, pre-eclampsia and eclampsia, bleeding in the antepartum period, fetal growth restriction, and cervical insufficiency. Risk factors for preterm birth are listed in Table 6-1. A causal association between these risk factors and preterm labor is difficult to assess because many women with preterm labor do not have preterm birth, and many of those who do have preterm labor go on to have full-term births.

> ### CLINICAL PEARL
> *Women with a history of preterm labor may benefit from progesterone supplementation, if initiated between 16 and 20 weeks of gestation (2).*

ACUTE MANAGEMENT AND WORKUP

The key to successfully managing preterm labor is early recognition. This allows for a coordinated effort from the labor and delivery team to maximize the conditions that improve fetal survival.

TABLE 6-1
Risk Factors for Preterm Labor[a]

Stress: Personal and Occupational
- Single; low socioeconomic status
- Anxiety, depression, life events
- Abdominal surgery during pregnancy
- Physical exertion, upright posture
- Use of industrial machines

Infection
- Sexually transmitted infections
- Pyelonephritis, appendicitis, pneumonia
- Bacteriuria
- Periodontal disease

Excessive or Impaired Uterine Distention
- Multiple gestation
- Polyhydramnios
- Uterine anomaly or fibroids
- Diethylstilbestrol

Placental Pathology
- Placenta previa
- Abruption
- Vaginal bleeding

Miscellaneous Factors
- Previous preterm delivery
- Substance abuse, smoking
- Age <18 or >40 years
- African American race
- Low BMI, weight gain
- Inadequate prenatal care
- Anemia (hemoglobin <10 g/dL)
- Excessive uterine contractility
- Low level of education
- Genotype

Fetal Factors
- Congenital anomaly
- Growth restriction
- Previous infant with SIDS

[a]BMI, body mass index; SIDS, sudden infant death syndrome.

The First 15 Minutes

When you initially assess someone for preterm labor, it is important to review her past medical history, including her obstetric history. It is then important to work on assessing the situation for the safety of the mother and the baby. Be sure you perform the following tasks:

1. *Determine the mother's vital signs.* Are the mother's vital signs stable? Is she having vaginal bleeding, is it excessive, causing signs and symptoms of anemia? Is she in pain?

2. *Determine the status of the fetus.* Are fetal hearts tones reassuring? Is the fetus in distress? Have the fetal membranes ruptured?

3. *Determine the frequency and strength of the contractions.* What is the contraction pattern and what is the strength of the contractions? Are the contractions coming frequently, infrequently, or continuously? Are they regular? Is the monitor picking them up? Are they palpating strongly or weakly?

4. *Obtain a history.* When did the contractions start? Have they increased in frequency or duration? What was the patient doing? Has she had recent intercourse or vaginal bleeding? Has she been eating and drinking? Have there been any problems in the pregnancy thus far? Are there any abnormalities in the placenta or its location? What is the exact gestational age of the fetus?

5. *Perform a pelvic exam.* You can do this via a sterile speculum exam. First, you should obtain a swab for fetal fibronectin, as this test is less accurate if there has been any prior cervical manipulation (e.g., previous exam, intercourse, vaginal bleeding). Next, rule in or out the rupture of membranes, perform tests for gonorrhea and chlamydia, and obtain a specimen for wet mount preparation. Then obtain a rectovaginal group B streptococcal culture. Finally, if there are no contraindications, you can check the cervix.

Initial Assessment

Any diagnosis of preterm labor includes confirmation that the cervix has changed. Once cervical dilation or effacement has been documented, perform a transvaginal ultrasound to measure cervical length. This can help triage the level of concern for preterm birth. Obviously, if the mother or fetus is not stable, action toward stabilization or delivery needs to be taken.

Admission Criteria and Level of Care Criteria

Once the patient has been deemed stable, a transvaginal ultrasound can be performed. Some evidence exists to stratify patient's relative risk of preterm delivery based on cervical length (Table 6-2).

Option 1: Stable Condition

With rest and hydration, your patient's contractions can abate. If this occurs in the context of an otherwise reassuring exam, outpatient surveillance is reasonable.

Option 2: Fair Condition

Following assessment as previously described, with rest and hydration your patient's contractions continue. Her transvaginal cervical length or sterile

TABLE 6-2

Relative Risk of Preterm Delivery Based on Cervical Length

Cervical Length (mm)	Relative Risk of Preterm Delivery
<35	2.35
<30	3.79
<26	6.19
<22	9.49
<13	13.99

vaginal exams are more advanced, and thus treatment is warranted. Your patient should be admitted for the administration of glucocorticoids, for tocolysis, and for bed rest. Neonatologists should be available for discussion with the patient, and the fetal position should be assessed to address the most appropriate mode of delivery, should delivery become imminent.

Option 3: Critical Condition

Following assessment as previously described, the patient has continued contractions and a repeat cervical exam shows that delivery is imminent. At this point, the neonatal pediatricians need to be involved in the patient's care. If the fetus is vertex, a vaginal delivery is the preferred method of delivery. If the fetus is breech, you should counsel the patient on the risks and benefits of a breech delivery in a preterm fetus. If transverse, the preferred delivery method is cesarean section.

The First Few Hours

After determining the acuity of your patient's condition, the next step is to determine a management plan. Typically, rest and hydration are therapies performed as the management is taking place. In the absence of imminent delivery, you can wait as each of your lab results come back. Continue to monitor contraction strength and frequency. Evidence of progression will necessitate admission for the administration of glucocorticoids, for tocolysis, and for observation.

History

Key points to assess in the initial history include obvious issues like past medical and surgical histories as well as a detailed obstetric and gynecologic history. For example, has the patient had any cervical procedures, or does she have any history of preterm birth? Signs of preterm labor can be very nonspecific. Symptoms like mild cramping, constant low back pain, mild irregular contractions, and vaginal spotting are often present in various times of pregnancy without issues.

Another key issue includes confirming gestational age. Once a fetus has reached 34 weeks of gestation, treatment for the inhibition of labor is not undertaken, as the perinatal morbidity and mortality are thought to be too low to justify the maternal and fetal complications.

Physical Examination

One should minimize the number of cervical exams performed in an attempt to reduce the chances of rupturing membranes or inducing an infection.

Labs and Tests to Consider

Important first steps are the collection of cervical samples for fetal fibronectin, a wet-mount preparation, and cultures for genital infections. Basic diagnostic labs to perform include a complete blood count with differential. This allows assessment of hemodynamic status and infection. A urinalysis is obtained to diagnose a reversible, infectious cause of preterm labor.

CLINICAL PEARL

The absence of fetal fibronectin from a cervicovaginal swab will reliably predict that the pregnancy will continue for another 2 weeks. This test is useful in women experiencing preterm contractions between 24 and 34 weeks of gestation.

Imaging

Once the patient is stabilized, a detailed ultrasound scan should be performed. Ultrasound can provide data for assessment of the fetus. Key things to look for in an ultrasound include evidence of fetal viability and the absence of any fetal anomalies. Any ultrasound should assess for placental location and signs of insufficiency.

Treatment

The goal of the treatment of preterm labor is to identify the stimulus that initiated the process of cervical change. Once you identify the stimulus, it should be corrected, such as administering antibiotics for infection and fluid for dehydration. Tocolytics are a large part of any initial treatment. Most often, tocolytics are given with the intent of delaying delivery by at least 48 hours so that glucocorticoids can be given to the mother. Steroid therapy given prior to delivery has been shown to reduce the complications of preterm birth. Other instances in which tocolytics to delay delivery can have maximal effect is allowing for transportation of the mother to a facility that allows the level of critical care needed for a preterm delivery.

CLINICAL PEARL

There are two main reasons tocolytic therapy is administered to women experiencing preterm labor: (1) to attempt to delay delivery by 48 hours for the administration of glucocorticoids, and (2) to allow for maternal transport to a facility that can handle a premature infant.

There are obvious situations in which tocolysis is not indicated. These can be summarized by assessing if the fetus or mother is better off if delivery is imminent. Situations like this include maternal hemorrhage with maternal hemodynamic instability, chorioamnionitis, severe growth restriction, or severe pre-eclampsia, eclampsia, or nonreassuring fetal status. In the situation of lethal fetal anomalies or fetal demise, the treatment of preterm labor is not undertaken.

Tocolysis takes the form of administering beta-adrenergic receptor agonists (terbutaline), calcium channel blockers (nifedipine), and nonsteroidal anti-inflammatory drugs (indomethacin). Magnesium is no longer the standard of care for tocolysis.

Terbutaline causes myometrial relaxation by increasing adenyl cyclase, which activates protein kinase and the phosphorylation of intracellular proteins. This leads to a drop in intracellular free calcium, which interferes with the activity of myosin light chain kinase, thereby interfering with the interaction of actin and myosin, and thus myometrial contractility. Eventually, cells become desensitized to the effects of terbutaline. Beta-adrenergic receptor agonist tocolytic therapy has been shown to decrease the number of women giving birth within 48 hours. Common maternal side effects include tachycardia, palpitations, hypokalemia, hyperglycemia, and lower blood pressure. It should not be used on women with a history of cardiac disease, myasthenia gravis, or poorly controlled hyperthyroidism or diabetes.

Calcium channel blockers, like beta-adrenergic receptor agonists, inhibit calcium-dependent myosin light chain kinase phosphorylation and thus result in myometrial relaxation. A meta-analysis of trials comparing calcium channel blockers to other tocolytics did not show them to significantly reduce the risk of birth within 48 hours, but they did show a reduction in the risk of birth within 7 days. When compared directly with beta-adrenergic receptor agonists, calcium channel blockers did significantly decrease risk of preterm birth within 48 hours of initiating treatment. Maternal side effects are a consequence of peripheral vasodilation and can include nausea, flushing, headache, dizziness, and palpitations. The primary fetal concern centers on maintaining good uterine and umbilical blood flow. Calcium channel blockers should not be used by women with ventricular dysfunction or congestive heart failure.

The cyclooxygenase inhibitor indomethacin prevents the conversion of arachidonic acid to prostaglandins. Without prostaglandins, the formation of myometrial gap junctions is decreased. Limited trials exist to support the use of indomethacin as a tocolytic. However, the evidence is promising. The maternal side effects are those of prolonged use of nonsteroidal anti-inflammatory drugs, and the fetal side effects are premature constriction of the ductus arteriosus (usually not before 31 to 32 weeks) and oligohydramnios. These are typically a consequence of longer in utero exposure (>72 hours).

In the past, magnesium sulfate was used for tocolysis. Its mechanism of action is not known, and to date there is no evidence of significant reductions in preterm birth. Randomized trials of magnesium use to prevent fetal neurologic deficits showed either no long-term protective effect of magnesium or harm to the fetus from magnesium therapy in the mother. Toxicity risks for magnesium are profound and are related to serum concentration. They begin with loss of deep tendon reflexes, progress to respiratory paralysis, and then to cardiac arrest.

EXTENDED IN-HOSPITAL MANAGEMENT

Preterm labor is not a pathology well suited to extended in-hospital management. After the initial treatment with tocolysis and steroids, patients continue with inpatient observation more for the neonatal indication of preterm delivery. Inpatient management most often consists of bed rest and serial fetal assessment.

DISPOSITION

Discharge Goals

The arrest of preterm labor is the goal prior to discharge. Each case should be assessed individually, taking into account cervical dilation, length, and effacement. Most often, patients are not discharged prior to at least 28 weeks of gestation. At 28 weeks, you can assess the patient for possible discharge home, typically through assessing cervical length and dilation with attention given to temporal trends.

Outpatient Care

Once a patient has been found to have an arrest of preterm labor, she should continue with normal prenatal care, with additional cervical monitoring for any signs or symptoms of further preterm labor. This includes tocometry when contractions are present, the measurement of cervical lengths up to 34 weeks, and sterile cervical exams as necessary.

WHAT YOU NEED TO REMEMBER

- For the diagnosis of preterm labor, you must document cervical change.
- All attempts should be made to find a reversible cause of preterm labor.
- Tocolysis is of limited utility. If not contraindicated, it should be initiated to allow glucocorticoids to be given to achieve maximal fetal protective benefit and transport to a facility that will provide maximal support to the preterm neonate.
- Begin tocolysis with calcium channel blockers because of their low cost, ease of administration, efficacy, and the low frequency of side effects. For second-line treatment in patients at <32 weeks of gestation, consider indomethacin. For second-line treatment in pregnancies 32 to 34 weeks, consider beta-adrenergic receptor agonists.

REFERENCES

1. Hamilton BE, Martin JA, Ventura SJ. Births: Preliminary data for 2006. National vital statistics reports; vol. 56, no. 7. Hyattsville, MD: National Center for Health Statistics; 2007.
2. American College of Obstetricians and Gynecologists. ACOG committee opinion number 419: use of progesterone to reduce preterm birth. *Obstet Gynecol.* 2008;112:963–965.

SUGGESTED READINGS

American College of Obstetricians and Gynecologists. ACOG practice bulletin number 31: assessment of risk factors for preterm birth. *Obstet Gynecol.* 2001;98:709–716.

American College of Obstetricians and Gynecologists. ACOG practice bulletin number 43: management of preterm labor. *Obstet Gynecol.* 2003;101:1039–1047.

Cunningham G, Leveno KL, Bloom SL, et al. Obstetrical hemorrhage. In: *Williams Obstetrics.* 22nd ed. New York, NY: McGraw-Hill; 2005:809–855.

Swamy GK, Østbye T, Skjærven R. Association of preterm birth with long-term survival, reproduction, and next-generation JAMA, Preterm Birth. *JAMA.* 2008; 299(12):1429–1436.

March of Dimes Peristats. http://www.marchofdimes.com/peristats. Accessed October 27, 2008.

Preterm Premature Rupture of Membranes

THE PATIENT ENCOUNTER

A 26-year-old woman (G2P1) at 32 weeks, 4 days of gestation walks into the triage area complaining of feeling a "gush" of fluid escape while she was sleeping. She thought she involuntarily urinated, but noticed that the fluid was continuously leaking after the initial gush. She denies any lower abdominal pain or vaginal bleeding, and she endorses fetal movement.

OVERVIEW

Definition

The rupture of membranes before the onset of labor that occurs before 37 weeks of gestation is referred to as preterm premature rupture of membranes (pPROM). While a patient with *term* premature rupture of membranes (PROM) who is not in labor may proceed to delivery, *preterm* rupture requires a more thorough evaluation to decide between expectant management and delivery. The goal in managing these patients is prolonging the pregnancy to avoid fetal complications while minimizing risks to the mother.

Pathophysiology

Membranes rupture for a variety of reasons, but the reason why is not always clear for each individual patient. Intra-amniotic infection is commonly associated with PROM, in addition to mechanical shearing forces created by uterine contractions. For the fetus, the complications related to prematurity carry the most significant risks. Respiratory distress is reported as the most common source of morbidity, but others include neonatal infections, intraventricular hemorrhage, and necrotizing enterocolitis. There is also a 1% to 2% risk of fetal demise, usually secondary to sepsis and cord accidents (1).

Epidemiology

Preterm PROM affects 1.7% of pregnancies versus 8% at term. By the time most patients present, 75% are already in labor and 10% deliver in 48 hours (2).

Etiology

PPROM is attributed to certain risk factors. Women with a prior preterm birth, a short cervical length, as well as current preterm labor symptoms are at risk for having preterm PROM. Additional factors include low socioeconomic status, bleeding, low body mass index, connective tissue disorders, cigarette smoking, cervical conization, pulmonary disease, uterine overdistention, and amniocentesis. All patients receiving amniocentesis should be counseled about the 1% to 1.2% risk of pPROM (3). The outcome of post-amniocentesis PROM, however, is better than that after spontaneous preterm PROM. In many patients, the membranes reseal with restoration of normal amniotic fluid volume.

ACUTE MANAGEMENT AND WORKUP

The two goals in the acute management of PROM are to determine whether the membranes are actually ruptured and whether the patient is in labor.

The First 15 Minutes

Initial management includes a thorough history with a few focused key points, such as the exact time of rupture and the color of the fluid, the presence of contractions, and fever at home.

Initial Assessment

When you encounter a patient with potential PROM, you must first confirm that the membranes have actually ruptured. You can initially assess the patient by performing a sterile speculum exam looking for ferning, amniotic fluid pooling, or change in nitrazine. If those are equivocal, you can consider an abdominal ultrasound to look at the amniotic fluid index within the uterus.

Admission Criteria and Level of Care Criteria

If you do confirm that a patient has experienced a true PROM, the patient will need to be admitted and observed in the hospital until delivery. The decision to induce labor or expectantly manage the pregnancy will depend on the gestational age at the time of rupture and the fetal assessment. If the patient is beyond 34 weeks of gestation or there are any signs of chorioamnionitis, labor is traditionally induced.

The First Few Hours

The first few hours of the assessment are geared toward ensuring that the patient does not go into preterm labor.

History

After you obtain an exact history related to the timing of the rupture, the next part of the history should focus on the risk factors that may have precipitated the PROM.

Physical Examination

Once the history suggests the likely diagnosis, fetal assessment and sterile vaginal examinations are next in the management algorithm. You should closely observe the patient's vital signs—specifically, fever and tachycardia. A sterile speculum exam is performed to evaluate for fluid accumulation or "pooling" in the vagina. If you do not initially see any fluid, you can ask the patient to cough or bear down as this may produce fluid from the os. The cervix should be visually inspected for visual dilatation, in lieu of a digital exam. Digital exams are typically avoided to decrease the chance of infection. The presence of blood should also be evaluated during the sterile speculum exam as it may indicate cervical change or even abruption.

Labs and Tests to Consider

Ultrasonography can also be used as a guiding tool for diagnosis by assessing the amnionic fluid volume as well as the presenting part. Caution is advised because a woman who has clearly ruptured clinically may still have a normal amnionic fluid volume. Additional methods of diagnosis include testing the pH of the vaginal fluid. Normal vaginal pH ranges between 4.5 and 5.5; amnionic fluid, however, will be more alkaline, in the range of 7.0 to 7.5. Another method is the use of the indicator nitrazine paper that undergoes a color reaction when the pH is >6.5. False-positive findings do occur when there is coexistent semen, blood, or bacterial vaginosis. The other laboratory test is detection of ferning of the vaginal fluid on a microscope slide (Fig. 7-1).

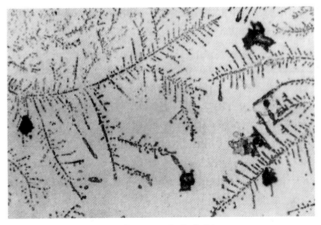

FIGURE 7-1: Ferning pattern from amniotic fluid.

> ### CLINICAL PEARL
>
> *The three tests that can help confirm the diagnosis of pPROM are change in nitrazine, ferning of the vaginal fluid, and pooling of amniotic fluid in the vagina.*

EXTENDED IN-HOSPITAL MANAGEMENT

Once pPROM has been established, the patient is monitored in the labor unit for fetal heart rate and uterine activity surveillance. The physician should decide whether the patient is in active labor, or if there are any indications for delivery such as chorioamnionitis or fetal distress.

Option 1: Greater than 34 Weeks of Gestation, Laboring and Nonlaboring Patients

If a patient is >34 weeks of gestation, labor is typically induced using oxytocin. Group B streptococcal prophylaxis is administered and corticosteroids are not recommended.

Option 2: Less than 34 Weeks of Gestation, Laboring Patients

If the patient appears to be in labor, as evidenced by her sterile speculum exam or contraction pattern, observation in labor and delivery is warranted. Intrapartum surveillance is continued because variable decelerations can occur with occult umbilical cord compression. The uterine activity aids in monitoring the labor pattern while avoiding frequent digital exams. If the patient is <32 weeks of gestation, corticosteroids are administered in order to reduce the prematurity complications. Antibiotics are also given for intrapartum prophylaxis from group B streptococcus unless the patient has a negative screen for group B streptococcus. The patient's labor course is monitored and augmented once she enters active labor (>4 cm dilation and >75% effacement). You should discuss the case with your neonatologist and ensure that he or she is present for resuscitation after delivery.

Option 3: Less than 34 Weeks Gestation, Nonlaboring Patients

A nonlaboring patient who is <34 weeks of gestation is admitted to the hospital and managed expectantly. She is usually put on pelvic and bed rest. You should administer a course of corticosteroids to reduce the neonatal morbidity associated with prematurity. Generally, a 7-day course of parenteral and oral therapy with ampicillin or amoxicillin and erythromycin is recommended to prolong pregnancy and reduce infectious and prematurity morbidity (1) (Table 7-1).

TABLE 7-1

Medications Commonly Used in the Management of Premature Rupture of Membranes[a]

Treatment Class	Medication and Duration	Indication
Antibiotics	Erythromycin × 10 d	Prolong pregnancy
	Amoxicillin-clavulonaic acid × 10 d	Prolonged pregnancy at 7 days but increased risk of necrotizing enterocolitis
	Ampicillin and erythromycin IV × 48 hours, amoxicillin and erythromycin × 5 d	Decreased likelihood of chorioamniotic and prolong delivery for up to 3 weeks
Steroids	Betamethasone 12 mg IM q24h × 2 doses	—
	Dexamethasone 6 mg IM q12h × 4 doses	—
GBS Prophylaxis	Penicillin G 5 mU IV load, then 2.5 mU IV q4h until delivery	—
	Ampicillin 2 g IV load, then 1 g IV q4h until delivery	—
	Clindamycin 900 mg IV q8h until delivery or erythromycin 500 mg IV q6h until delivery	If PCN allergic

[a]IV, intravenously; IM, intramuscularly; GBS, group B streptococcus; PCN, penicillin.

Tocolytics are primarily administered to allow for a full course of antenatal corticosteroids.

In the hospital, you should closely monitor for signs of chorioamnionitis and fetal well-being. Daily rounds should be attentive to vital signs as well as fundal tenderness or foul-smelling leaking fluid. If chorioamnionitis is diagnosed, the risk of prolonging pregnancy does not outweigh the increased infectious and neonatal morbidity, and the induction of labor with broad-spectrum antibiotics is indicated.

If the patient does not go into labor and has no other indications for delivery (chorioamnionitis, fetal distress) while in the hospital, the decision to deliver is usually based on provider and institutional preferences. Labor induction is warranted between 32 and 34 weeks of gestation, after confirming fetal lung maturity (4). If not, expectant management is continued. Delivery is generally recommended after 34 weeks of gestation because of the increased risk of chorioamnionitis and because corticosteroids are not recommended beyond this point (5).

CLINICAL PEARL

If your patient has experienced pPROM before 34 weeks, 7 days of antibiotics (ampicillin and erythromycin intravenously × 48 hours, amoxicillin and erythromycin orally × 5 days) will prolong the latent phase of labor for up to 3 weeks.

DISPOSITION

Discharge Goals

Postpartum social work and chaplain services can help the patient cope with the difficulties of caring for a preterm infant. Communication with the pediatrics team and the patient is important, especially if the infant's condition is concerning.

Outpatient Care

The patient's mental well-being should be evaluated at the postpartum visits as well, whether the infant has been discharged home or is still in the hospital, as this may place a lot of stress on a family. Patients with pPROM should also be counseled that a recurrence risk between 16% and 32% is applicable to their future pregnancies (1).

WHAT YOU NEED TO REMEMBER

- The initial evaluation of a patient with suspected pPROM must include a sterile speculum examination, looking for signs of fluid pooling, nitrazine changes, and ferning.
- An abdominal ultrasound in the setting of an equivocal examination is helpful. Not only can you estimate the amniotic fluid index but you can also confirm whether the fetus position is vertex or breech.
- Corticosteroids should be administered before 32 weeks of gestation to decrease the neonatal morbidity associated with prematurity.
- Indications for proceeding with an induction of a premature fetus after rupture of membranes includes evidence of chorioamnionitis, documentation of fetal lung maturity, and the spontaneous onset of labor.

REFERENCES

1. American College of Obstetricians and Gynecologists. ACOG practice bulletin number 80: premature rupture of membranes. *Obstet Gynecol.* 2007;109:1007–1019.
2. Cunningham G, Leveno KJ, Bloom SL, et al. Preterm birth. In: *Williams Obstetrics.* 22nd ed. New York, NY: McGraw-Hill; 2005:855–881.
3. Eddleman K, Malone F, Sullivan L, et al. Pregnancy loss rates after mid-trimester amniocentesis. *Obstet Gynecol.* 2006;108:1067–1072.
4. American College of Obstetricians and Gynecologists. ACOG practice bulletin number 97: fetal lung maturity. *Obstet Gynecol.* 2008;112:717–726.
5. American College of Obstetricians and Gynecologists. ACOG committee opinion number 402: antenatal corticosteroid therapy for fetal maturation. *Obstet Gynecol.* 2008;111:805–807.

SUGGESTED READINGS

Mercer B. Preterm Premature Rupture of the Membranes: Current Approaches to Evaluation and Management. *Obstet Gynecol Clin North Am.* 2005;32(3):411–428.
Mercer BM, Miodovnik M, Thurnau GR, et al. Antibiotic therapy for reduction of infant morbidity after preterm premature rupture of the membranes: a randomized controlled trial. *JAMA.* 1997;278:989–995.

CHAPTER

8

Postpartum Hemorrhage

👥 THE PATIENT ENCOUNTER

You are emergently called by the nurse in labor and delivery room 5 to evaluate a patient for heavy bleeding approximately 1 hour following an uncomplicated spontaneous vaginal delivery. The patient is a 28-year-old woman (P5035) who just gave birth to a live, vigorous male infant weighting 4,200 g. Upon arrival, the patient reports that she felt a sudden gush of blood "down there" and now feels dizzy.

OVERVIEW

Definition

Postpartum hemorrhage is generally defined as >500-mL blood loss following a vaginal delivery and >1,000-mL blood loss following a cesarean section (1). The majority of cases of postpartum hemorrhage occur within the first 24 hours following delivery, and each is classified as "primary" or "early." Those cases occurring later than 24 hours following delivery but prior to 6 weeks postpartum are defined as "secondary" or "late." This chapter will focus on the causes of postpartum hemorrhage and medical versus surgical management options.

Pathophysiology

During pregnancy, maternal blood volume expands an average of 40% to 50% and red blood cell mass increases 20% to 30%. These changes aid in protecting both mother and fetus from hypotension related to the vasodilation associated with pregnancy, and helps in protecting the mother from hemorrhage in the postpartum period (2).

Epidemiology

Despite the changes previously noted, postpartum hemorrhage is the most common cause of maternal death worldwide, with an estimated 14 million women experiencing deliveries complicated by postpartum hemorrhage each year (3,4).

Etiology

Primary postpartum hemorrhage is most commonly caused by uterine atony, or failure of the uterus to adequately contract following delivery.

Additional etiologies include retained placental fragments, undetected lower genital tract lacerations, uterine inversion, uterine rupture, or defects in coagulation (2).

Secondary postpartum hemorrhage is often related to uterine atony that may be associated with infection, subinvolution of the placental bed, or retained products of conception (5). In addition, a late postpartum hemorrhage may represent the first sign of a hereditary coagulopathy, such as von Willebrand disease.

Risk factors for primary and secondary postpartum hemorrhage include the following (6,7): **Factors increasing risk for uterine atony:** overdistended uterus (polyhydramnios, multiple fetuses, large fetus), exhausted uterine musculature (rapid labor, prolonged labor, oxytocin or prostaglandin administration), anesthetic agents, history of uterine atony, high parity, or chorioamnionitis

- **Abnormal placentation:** placental abruption, placenta accrete, increta, or percreta
- **Trauma during labor and delivery:** episiotomy, vacuum or forceps delivery, or cesarean delivery
- **Factors increasing risk for uterine rupture:** high parity, prior uterine surgery, intrauterine manipulation, or uterine hyperstimulation
- **Low maternal blood volume:** severe pre-eclampsia, eclampsia, or small women
- **Coagulation defects:** associated with prolonged retention of a dead fetus, amniotic fluid embolism, sepsis, massive transfusion, anticoagulation therapy, severe intravascular hemolysis, severe preeclampsia, eclampsia, or hereditary coagulopathies
- **Other:** Asian, Hispanic or Native American ancestry; obesity; history of postpartum hemorrhage

ACUTE MANAGEMENT AND WORKUP

A postpartum hemorrhage may present as a sudden downpour of hemorrhage or as a constant leakage. In addition, the patient's blood pressure and pulse may demonstrate only mild alterations until an excessive amount of bleeding has occurred. Avoidance of morbidity depends on a high clinical index of suspicion and vigilance.

The First 15 Minutes

Given that approximately 500 mL/min of blood flows through the intervillous space, prompt intervention is essential.

Initial Assessment

The first thing to realize in the event of a postpartum hemorrhage is that blood loss in large amounts can cause some amount of frenzy and anxiety in the labor and delivery room. The number one rule is to remain calm and perform a focused history and physical exam:

1. Ask the patient how she is feeling. Is she alert and oriented? Is she responding appropriately to your questions?
2. What are the patient's vital signs? Has she become hypotensive or tachycardic? Is she febrile (temperature ≥38.0°C [100.4°F])?
3. Perform a pelvic exam. Inspect the perineum externally to look for active vaginal bleeding. Start bimanual massage: Perform a bimanual examination using your dominant hand to remove clots from the vagina and lower uterine segment, and the other hand to simultaneously massage the uterine fundus abdominally.
4. Does the patient have intravenous (IV) access? If not, insert at least one large-bore IV line. Run normal saline or lactated Ringers at 125 mL/h to start, and bolus IV fluids if the patient is hypotensive or tachycardic. Confirm that at least 20 U of oxytocin is in 1 L of fluid to assist with myometrial contractions and vasoconstriction.
5. Reassess the patient: Has the bleeding stopped? Is the uterine fundus firm and near the level of the umbilicus? Are the patient's vital signs still stable?

Admission Criteria and Level of Care Criteria

The next step is to determine the patient's condition in the labor and delivery room.

Option 1: Stable Condition

Following bimanual massage, the patient's vital signs are stable and active vaginal bleeding has stopped: Proceed with further monitoring in the labor and delivery room, with or without medical treatment.

Option 2: Fair Condition

Following bimanual massage, the patient's vital signs are stable, but she continues to have intermittent active vaginal bleeding during which time the uterine fundus becomes soft: Start medical treatment.

Option 3: Critical Condition

Following bimanual massage, the patient has continued, active vaginal bleeding that is primarily bright red and continues to saturate through pads and sheets, with or without tachycardia and hypotension: Start medical treatment immediately and repeat a pelvic exam with a speculum to visualize the entire vagina and cervix. Reinspect the placenta to rule out retained tissue. Start a second IV and confirm that blood products are immediately available if needed. If the patient remains unstable, transfer her to the operating room in preparation for surgical management if needed.

The First Few Hours

After determining your patient's condition, the next step is to make a plan for management as previously outlined. Rapid assessment of the patient's stability and response to therapy is critical.

History

Throughout the resuscitative process, periodic review of the patient's response to earlier therapy is essential. Many times, an assistant can be assigned to monitor the patient's ongoing blood loss. Include the anesthesiologist early in the intervention cycle as he or she may help facilitate volume replacement.

- Make the anesthesiologist aware of the patient's condition.
- Insert two large-bore IV catheters.
- Send STAT complete blood count, international normalized ratio/partial thromboplastin time. Make sure the patient has an active type and screen and call the blood bank to put at least two units of blood on hold.

Physical Examination

A bimanual examination should be performed to assess the fundal height, uterine tone, and presence of clots or placental products at the level of the internal os. In addition, the patient should be assessed for signs of impending hemorrhagic shock.

Labs and Tests to Consider

The main labs to order in this scenario are a complete blood count, prothrombin time/international normalized ratio/partial thromboplastin time, and an active type and screen. It is helpful to have an assistant personally call the blood bank to confirm the availability of blood products.

Imaging

If retained placental products are high in the differential diagnosis, a bedside abdominal ultrasound is easy to perform and is noninvasive. Imaging may provide insight into the amount of uterine products and may alert the obstetrician to consider an emergent suction dilation and curettage.

Treatment

There are both medical and surgical management options. You should always start with medical treatment and move to surgical options if medical treatment fails. Table 8-1 provides common medical treatment options.

CLINICAL PEARL

When faced with a postpartum hemorrhage, remember that methergine is contraindicated in patients with hypertension (pre-eclampsia or chronic hypertension) and Hemabate is contraindicated in patients with reactive airway disease.

TABLE 8-1
Medical Management of Postpartum Hemorrhage[a]

Medication	Dosage	Mechanism	Contraindications
Pitocin (oxytocin)	20 U in 500 mL saline @ 200 mL/h Or 10 U IM if no IV access (can also add 20 U to 1,000 mL NS and run @ 125 mL/h for 24 h postpartum)	Binds to receptors in the myometrium to induce uterine contractions	No contraindications Can have an antidiuretic effect at very high doses and result in volume overload. In addition, can cause serious hypotension
Methergine (methylergonovine maleate)	0.2 mg IM/IV (can give additional 0.2 mg PO q6–8h × 24–48 h following delivery)	Semisynthetic ergot alkaloid: causes a sustained tetanic effect on smooth muscle of the uterus	Cannot give to patients with HTN or Raynaud phenomenon Can cause N/V Interacts with macrolide antibiotics

| Hemabate (carboprost tromethamine) | 0.25 mg/1 amp IM or given directly in myometrium (can give q15–90 min × 8 doses) | Prostaglandin F2 alpha: causes smooth muscle contraction | Cannot give to patients with asthma or active renal, hepatic, or cardiac disease Can cause N/V/D; can increase body temp |
| Cytotec (misoprostol) | 600–800 mcg PR | Prostaglandin E1 analog | Use with caution in patientswith renal or cardiac disease |

[a]IM, intramuscularly; IV, intravenously; NS, normal saline; HTN, hypertension; PO, by mouth; N/V/D, nausea/vomiting/diarrhea; PR, per rectum.

If medical treatment fails and the patient continues to have active vaginal hemorrhage, additional measures are required. At this point, it is reasonable to move the patient back to the operating room for further evaluation. If the patient's vital signs have become unstable, the operating room provides a more controlled environment where the anesthesiology team can provide fluid and blood product resuscitation and prepare for a surgical procedure if needed. While in the operating room, the patient can also be properly positioned and receive adequate anesthesia to look for any previously missed vaginal or cervical lacerations.

An initial step to slow uterine bleeding is to tamponade the uterine cavity with packing. The uterus can be packed with dry lap sponges in order to apply direct pressure to the bleeding uterine cavity and to tamponade bleeding vessels. A similar effect may be achieved by inserting a balloon apparatus into the uterine cavity. There are specific balloon devices that have been constructed for this purpose, or one or more 30-mL Foley catheters can be used with similar outcomes. Once the balloon or catheter is inserted, it is then inflated to apply direct pressure against the uterine wall.

If uterotonic medical management in combination with packing fails to slow uterine bleeding, several surgical techniques can be implemented. If an exploratory laparotomy becomes necessary, a vertical midline incision is recommended to provide optimal exposure of the abdominal and pelvic cavities.

- *Uterine Curettage*. If retained products of conception are suspected, a uterine curettage can be performed with a large banjo curette. This should be performed under ultrasound guidance given the high risk of uterine perforation associated with this procedure and the gravid uterus.
- *O'Leary Uterine Artery Ligation*. The uterine artery and vein are located at the level of the lower uterine segment, and are ligated by passing 0-vicryl suture 2 to 3 cm medial to the vessels in the uterus, through the myometrium, and out lateral to the vessels through the broad ligament. Care should be taken to palpate and to avoid the ureter (Fig. 8-1).
- *B-Lynch Suture*. No. 2 chromic suture is passed through the inferior and left lateral aspect of the lower uterine segment, up through the superior aspect of the uterine incision, and is then passed over the uterine fundus in an anterior-to-posterior fashion. The suture is then passed from the posterior uterus into and through the uterine cavity to the right. It is then brought back over the uterine fundus in a posterior-to-anterior fashion, through the superior aspect of the uterine incision and out the inferior aspect. The needle is cut off and the suture ends are tied to compress the uterus.
- *Hypogastric (Internal Iliac) Artery Ligation*
- *Uterine Artery Embolization*. Used only in the case of a stable patient with persistent uterine bleeding. Embolization is performed by an interventional radiologist under radiographic guidance (Fig. 8-2).

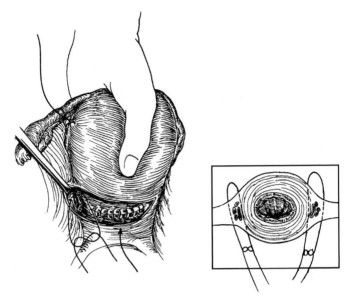

FIGURE 8-1: O'Leary uterine artery ligation.

- *Hysterectomy.* Hysterectomy is performed only after more conservative measures have failed. The pelvic anatomy may be grossly distorted by the gravid uterus and pelvic congestion. Extra care must the taken to avoid the ureters bilaterally. In the case of a placenta percreta, in which surrounding bowel or bladder may be involved, a gynecologic oncologist, general surgeon, or urologist should be present at the time of the procedure.

EXTENDED IN-HOSPITAL MANAGEMENT

Following medical or surgical management of postpartum hemorrhage, the patient's vital signs are monitored hourly and then every 4 hours if they remain stable. A pad count is used to monitor the amount of vaginal bleeding the patient continues to have. Fundal checks are employed to assure that the uterine fundus is firm and near or below the level of the umbilicus. Serial hematocrit levels may be drawn and blood transfusion should be considered with symptomatic anemia (i.e., chest pain, shortness of breath, dizziness), or with a hematocrit level below 20%.

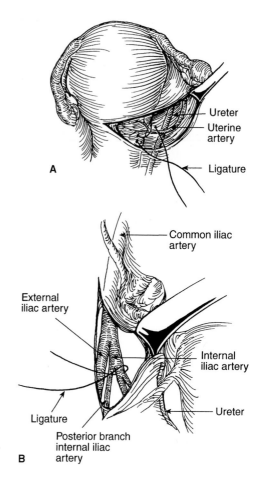

FIGURE 8-2: Hypogastric artery ligation.

DISPOSITION

Discharge Goals

After resolution of the acute phase of hemorrhage, the goal is to monitor for any evidence of a late hemorrhage and to confirm the patient's ability to perform the activities of daily living necessary to take care of a newborn while recovering.

- Vital signs should demonstrate that the patient is hemodynamically stable.
- Hematocrit levels should remain stable.
- Vaginal bleeding should decrease to normal lochia (i.e., moderate-to-heavy menses), and should continue to improve on a daily basis. Patients

should be cautioned that bleeding might temporarily increase with breast-feeding.

Outpatient Care

Conservative therapy with oral iron supplementation is sufficient for women to return to their baseline hematocrit. Outpatient care should include the following:

- An outpatient visit 4 to 6 weeks following delivery
- A physical exam, including a speculum and bimanual exam performed to ascertain normal uterine involution
- Counseling for patients about the increased risk of postpartum hemorrhage with future pregnancies
- In cases of late or secondary postpartum hemorrhage, a coagulopathy workup up may be considered.

 WHAT YOU NEED TO REMEMBER

- Postpartum hemorrhage is the most common cause of maternal death worldwide.
- Primary postpartum hemorrhage occurs within 24 hours following delivery and is most commonly caused by uterine atony.
- Secondary postpartum hemorrhage occurs between 24 hours and 6 weeks following delivery. Retained products of conception and maternal coagulopathy should be considered.
- Medical management aims at inducing uterine contraction.
- Postpartum hemorrhage can become a surgical emergency if medical management fails. Successful management depends on coordination between nursing staff and obstetric and anesthesia teams, and relies on IV access, fluid resuscitation, and procedure execution.

REFERENCES

1. Prendiville WJ, Elbourne D, McDonald S. Active versus expectant management in the third stage of labour. *Cochrane Database Syst Rev.* 2000;3:CD000007.
2. Gabbe SG, Niebyl JR, Simpson JL. *Obstetrics: Normal and Problem Pregnancies.* 4th ed. New York, NY: Churchill Livingstone; 2002:72–73.
3. Potts M, Hemmerling A. The worldwide burden of postpartum haemorrhage: policy development where inaction is lethal. *Int J Gynecol Obstet.* 2006;94:S116–S121.
4. World Health Organization. *Mother–Baby Package.* Geneva, Switzerland: World Health Organization; 1998.

5. Khong TY, Khong TK. Delayed postpartum hemorrhage: a morphologic study of causes and their relation to other pregnancy disorders. *Obstet Gynecol.* 1993;82: 17–22.
6. Herbert WNP, Zelop CM. American College of Obstetricians and Gynecologists practice bulletin number 76: postpartum hemorrhage. *Obstet Gynecol.* 2006;108: 1039–1048.
7. Cunningham G, Leveno KL, Bloom SL, et al. Obstetrical hemorrhage. In: *Williams Obstetrics.* 22nd ed. New York, NY: McGraw-Hill; 2005:809–854.

SUGGESTED READINGS

Hofmeyr GJ, Abdel-Aleem H, Abdel-Aleem MA. Uterine massage for preventing postpartum haemorrhage. *Cochrane Database Syst Rev.* 2008;(3):CD006431.
Oyelese Y, Scorza W, Mastrolia R, et al. Postpartum hemorrhage. *Obstet Gynecol Clin North Am* 2007;34(3):421–441.

Postpartum Fever

THE PATIENT ENCOUNTER

You are called by the emergency department nurse in charge of exam room 8. A 28-year-old woman (G2P2) on her fourth day after cesarean section has a fever of 38.5°C (101.3°F), a foul-smelling odor, and general malaise.

OVERVIEW

The term *postpartum fever* or *puerperal infection* applies to all the infectious processes that may be present following a vaginal or cesarean delivery. Historically, before antibiotics were used, puerperal infections were the principal cause of deaths of women who gave birth.

Definition

Postpartum fever is typically the initial sign of a postdelivery infection. Other symptoms, such as abdominal pain or a foul-odor vaginal discharge, may be present in conjunction with a postpartum fever.

Pathophysiology

Because of the broad nature of postpartum fevers, the exact pathophysiology is not known. What has been appreciated is that postpartum fevers are polymicrobial and respond well to broad-spectrum antibiotics.

Epidemiology

Postpartum infection is estimated to occur in 1% to 8% of all deliveries in the United States (1). Maternal deaths associated with infection range from 4% to 8%, or approximately 0.6 maternal deaths per 100,000 live births.

Etiology

The polymicrobial nature of postpartum infections makes identifying a single etiology difficult. The most common causes of a postpartum fever are summarized in Table 9-1.

Although a postpartum fever is not equivocally synonymous with an infection, an appreciation of the individual risk factors will heighten one's

TABLE 9-1

Summary of the Most Common Causes of Postpartum Fever

Site of Infection	Cause
Endometritis	The bacteria responsible for uterine contamination and pelvic infections are anaerobic and aerobic bacteria, which normally reside in the bowel, vagina, perineum, and cervix. The uterus is usually sterile until the rupture of the amniotic sac, labor or instrumentation is present. Cesarean deliveries increase the risk by 85%.[a] In 90% of cases, the originating bacteria ascended from vagina.
Genital Tract Infections	In general, all genital tract infections will be polymicrobial, involving *Escherichia coli* and gram-positive cocci, *Bacteroides* and *Clostridium* species.
Urinary Tract Infections (UTIs)	The bacteria frequently involved in UTIs normally reside in the bowel flora, including *E. coli* (85% of all cases), *Klebsiella* spp, *Proteus* spp, *Staphylococcus* spp, and *Enterobacter* spp.
	Any form of instrumentation or urethral manipulation (Foley or Nelaton catheterization) increases the risk of acquisition of a UTI and the presence of biofilm on catheters, which increase bacteria colonization.
Thrombosis	Pregnant and postpartum women are very susceptible to thrombotic events. Pregnancy is known to induce a hypercoagulable state secondary to increased levels of coagulation factors.

TABLE 9-1
Summary of the Most Common Causes of Postpartum Fever (Continued)

Site of Infection	Cause
	On the other hand, venous stasis in the pelvic veins during pregnancy can also induce thrombotic events. Septic pelvic thrombosis is observed in postpartum patients who may present with fever for more than 5 days even with correct treatment, (1:3,000 deliveries).[b] These cases, fortunately, are rare.
Perineal Cellulitis and Episiotomy Site Infections	*Staphylococcus* spp or *Streptococcus* spp and gram-negative organisms are responsible for the majority of cases. Fortunately only from 0.1%−2% of patients who had a vaginal tear or episiotomy will develop an infectious process.[b]
Mastitis	*Staphylococcus aureus* is the most frequently microorganism found in mastitis cases. Usually associated to the breastfeeding infant's mouth or throat, or mother skin.

[a]Anstey MT, Sheldon GW, Blyth JF. Infectious morbidity after cesarean section in private institution. *Am J Obstet Gynecol.* 1980;136:205–210.
[b]Mandell, Bennett, Dolin. *Principles and Practice of Infectious Diseases.* 6th ed. New York, NY: Churchill Livingstone; 2006.

index of suspicion. The risk factors a provider should inquire about during the initial assessment include the following:

• Obesity
• Poor nutritional status
• Human immunodeficiency virus
• Immunosuppression

- Poor prenatal care
- Vaginal infections
- Prolonged rupture of membranes
- Prolonged labor
- Cesarean section
- Premature rupture of membranes
- Frequent cervical examination
- Internal fetal monitoring devices
- Preexisting pelvic infection

> ### CLINICAL PEARL
>
> *Although infection tends to be the most common reason for postpartum fevers, don't forget noninfectious etiologies such as tissue ischemia, inflammation, thromboembolisms, epidurals, and even medications.*

ACUTE MANAGEMENT AND WORKUP

In the setting of an elevated temperature, the initial workup is critical for the correct diagnosis because the possibilities of an infectious source are numerous. An initial short and accurate history may orient you on the severity of the case. A good clinical evaluation and gathering the patient's history and risk factors will help narrow the diagnosis. Laboratory testing, radiology studies, and diagnostic laparoscopy are resources that are the most available in every clinic and will help diagnosis.

The First 15 Minutes

Fever and general malaise will typically be observed in patients with a postpartum fever. The first 15 minutes of contact are very important to create the right clinical setting to obtain vital signs and initial information, which will help in establishing a precise diagnosis. Quickly assess the patient's health status; if critically ill, intensive care resources should be employed until the patient is stable.

Initial Assessment

The first thing to realize when facing a patient with suspected postpartum fever is that although symptoms may appear to be mild, the degree of infection can be serious and can spread quickly, especially when cesarean sections are involved. It is important to verify that the patient is hemodynamically stable. Obtaining vital signs upon arrival will give you a sense of the general health status of your patient. Perform a focused history and physical exam:

1. Ask the patient how she is feeling. Evaluate if she is alert, is oriented to time and space, and is able to respond correctly to your questions.
2. What are the patient's vital signs? Is she febrile? Is she tachycardia? Is she breathing normally? What is her blood oxygen saturation? How is her blood pressure?
3. Start evaluating her abdomen.
   • Listen for bowel sounds with a stethoscope. Are they normal?
   • Look for signs of lower abdominal tenderness or peritoneal irritability. Is lower abdominal pain present? Look for signs of redness, a warm temperature, or fluid secretion on the c-section scar if present.
4. Evaluate her pelvis.
   • Perform a pelvic exam with emphasis placed on an adequate perineal assessment for infected episiotomies and purulent uterine drainage. If present, take cultures and Gram stain.
   • Perform a wet mount and a vaginal Ph measure, looking for evidence of bacterial vaginosis.
   • Perform a gentle bimanual exam. Remember that you are looking for signs of tenderness in her cervix, uterus, or adnexa, along with possible masses and pus collections. Gently move her cervix and uterus to the sides. Is pain present? Is it acute? Look for masses, enlarged ovaries, or uterine and/or general tenderness.
5. Evaluate her breasts.
   • Perform a thorough exam of her breasts because signs of tenderness and swelling, as well as temperature, color, and/or size changes, may be found in relation with a mastitis process. Take note of every positive sign and symptom.
6. Does the patient have an intravenous (IV) access? If not, start an IV access with normal saline solution or Ringer lactate infusing at 125 mL/h.
7. While starting the IV access, take blood samples for laboratory tests. See the section "Labs and Tests to Consider" later in the chapter for suggested laboratory tests to be ordered.
8. Keep the patient monitored at all times until a final diagnosis is achieved.

Admission Criteria and Level of Care Criteria

The next step is to determine the patient's condition and severity of illness.

Option 1: Stable Condition

A patient is considered to be in stable condition under the following circumstances: The patient has mild signs and symptoms, vital signs are stable or normal, the patient has no more than a mild fever (temperature <38°C [100.4°F]), and, in general, no clear evidence of an acute infectious process is present. Under these conditions, a short in-hospital stay or close outpatient evaluation may be considered.

Option 2: Fair Condition

A patient is considered to be in fair condition under the following circumstances: The patient has mild-to-severe signs and symptoms, vital signs are stable or normal, the patient has fever >38°C (100.4°F), and evidence of an acute infectious process is present. Under these conditions, in-hospital management with further radiologic and laboratory testing along with antibiotic treatment should be started.

Option 3: Critical Condition

A patient is considered to be in critical condition under the following circumstances: The patient has severe signs and symptoms as well as fever >38°C (100.4°F), and signs suggestive or septic shock (e.g., hypotension and tachycardia) are present. Under these conditions, the patient should be immediately hospitalized, with IV antibiotics and aggressive fluid resuscitation administered. Consider surgical management or wound debridement if signs of abscess or pelvic mass are present.

The First Few Hours

The first few hours are critical when a patient is hospitalized. As in every patient undergoing an acute infectious process, the risk of sepsis or septic shock should be considered, and the patient should be kept under strict monitoring and surveillance. It is mandatory to follow up on pending tests to confirm the severity of the disease. Remember to keep the patient and family members well informed at all times. Remember also that breastfeeding should be stopped until the severity of symptoms is resolved and breast milk safety for baby has been regained.

History

The patient history and course of the delivery are very important pieces of information when performing an evaluation of a patient with postpartum fever. Important aspects of the patient history that you should consider in your assessment include the following:

- Route of delivery (vaginal or cesarean section)
- Length of ruptured membranes and labor
- Patient symptomatology
- Wound drainage, including erythema from surgical incision or episiotomy sites
- Urinary symptoms such as dysuria, flank pain, and increased urinary frequency
- Upper respiratory symptoms, such as dyspnea, cough, and chest pain
- Fever and chills
- Purulent and foul-smelling lochia

- Abdominal pain
- Breast tenderness, engorgement, or erythema

Physical Examination

Your physical examination of the patient should focus on identifying the primary source of infection. A complete physical examination, focusing on the chest and abdomen, and including pelvic and breast examinations, is necessary (Table 9-2).

Labs and Tests to Consider

Labs and tests to consider include the following:

- Complete blood count, including observing for a leucocyte count of 14,000 or greater
- Complete blood biochemistry
- Blood cultures, if sepsis is suspected
- Urinalysis, with cultures and sensitivity tests
- Wound cultures, if appropriate
- Vaginal wet mount, observing the white blood count
- Erythrocyte sedimentation rate, observing for an elevated count
- C-reactive protein, observing for an elevated level
- Endometrial biopsy, observing for histologic evidence of endometritis
- Culdocentesis, observing for a positive test with purulent material
- Human immunodeficiency virus screening

Key Diagnostic Labs and Tests

The four most important diagnostic keys are the following:

1. Leukocytosis of 14,000 or more on complete blood count
2. Cultures
3. Gram stain
4. White blood count observed on vaginal wet mount

Imaging

Pelvic ultrasonography may be helpful in detecting a wound abscess, a pelvic abscess, or an infected hematoma. In some cases, a computed tomography scan of the abdomen/pelvis with and without contrast may be helpful if there is concurrent concern for pelvic and other nonabdominal/pelvic sources of the infection (e.g., appendicitis, colitis) (2). Breast ultrasound can be helpful in evaluating mastitis and possible abscess formation.

Treatment

Broad-spectrum antibiotic coverage is recommended given the polymicrobial nature of postpartum infections. Classic combinations for endometritis include clindamycin or metronidazole + aminoglucosides + ampicillin.

TABLE 9-2

Physical Examination Findings Associated with Postpartum Fever

Site of Infection	Findings on Physical Examination
Endometritis	• Lower abdominal pain on one or both sides of the abdomen, • Adnexal and/or parametrial pain triggered by a bimanual examination, • Temperature elevation >38.0°C (100.4°F) or more on one occasion or 37.7°C (99.9°F) on two occasions 6 h apart
Abnormal vaginal or uterine discharge	• Foul-smelling lochia without other evidence of infection • Group A beta-hemolytic streptococci associated with scanty odorless lochia
Wound infections	• Erythema • Edema • Tenderness • Discharge from wound or • Episiotomy site
Mastitis	• Frequently unilateral • Erythematous breasts • Tenderness • Engorged
Urinary infections	• Tenderness costovertebral angle • Elevated temperature • Dysuria • Urinary frequency
Respiratory infections	• Rales • Cough • Consolidation • Rhonchi
Thrombotic events	• Palpable pelvic veins • Tachycardia out of proportion in relation to fever. • Regional pain

This will provide adequate coverage until Gram stain and cultures confirm sensitivities. If clinical signs do not improve over the course of 48 hours, antibiotic modifications are appropriate (3). Treatment failures are associated with resistant bacteria, the presence of viral infection at the time, an infected hematoma, a pelvic abscess, a myometrial abscess, pelvic vein septic thrombosis, and drug-induced fever (4).

> ### CLINICAL PEARL
> *The treatment of postpartum fevers secondary to infections involve broad-spectrum antibiotics. A well-studied example is a combination of ampicillin, gentamicin, and clindamycin.*

EXTENDED IN-HOSPITAL MANAGEMENT

In cases of severe or acute postpartum fever, patients should be hospitalized until symptoms resolve completely and lab tests are back to normal. Often, to assure patient compliance with treatment, prolonged hospitalization is required. Follow up on culture results and adjust antibiotics based on bacteria identified and their sensitivities.

DISPOSITION
Discharge Goals

The patient can be discharged when the following criteria are met:

- Vital signs demonstrate that the patient is stable and that her fever has resolved.
- The patient's complete blood count leukocyte count has returned to normal.
- General symptoms have resolved.
- Abscess, surgical debridement, and/or wound infection have resolved.
- The patient is able to tolerate oral treatment.

Outpatient Care

Before resuming breast-feeding, the patient should receive counseling regarding breast-feeding. The patient should be instructed to abstain from sexual intercourse for at least 6 weeks or until the signs of uterine involution appear to be normal. A 2-week follow-up visit is required in order to evaluate the clinical resolution of symptoms.

WHAT YOU NEED TO REMEMBER

- Postpartum infection can be a life-threatening process.
- Postpartum fever can appear in 1% to 8% of all deliveries.
- The early detection and diagnosis of postpartum fever is key for recovery without sequelae.
- A thorough history and physical exam are necessary to make an accurate diagnosis.
- Cultures of the infection site are important for correct treatment.
- Labs and radiologic imaging can assist you in assessing the severity of disease.
- Broad-spectrum antibiotics are initially recommended.
- Follow-up should be arranged 2 weeks after treatment resolution and/or discharge.

REFERENCES

1. Yokoe DS, Christiansen CL, Johnson R, et al. Epidemiology of and surveillance for postpartum infections. *Emerg Infect Dis.* 2001;7(5):837–841.
2. Brown CE, Stettler RW, Twicler D, Cunningham FG. Puerperal septic pelvic thrombophlebitis: Incidence and response to heparin therapy. *Am J Obstet Gynecol.* 1999;181:143–148.
3. Martens MG, Faro S, Hammill H, et al. Ampicillin/sulbactam versus clindamycin/gentamycin in the treatment of postpartum endometritis. *South Med J.* 1990;83:408–413.
4. Witlin AG, Mercer BM, Sibai BM. Septic pelvic thrombophlebitis or refractory postpartum fever of undetermined etiology. *J Maternal Fetal Med.* 1996;5:335–358.

SUGGESTED READINGS

Anstey MT, Sheldon GW, Blyth JF. Infectious morbidity after cesarean section in private institution. *Am J Obstet Gynecol.* 1980;136:205–210.

Faro S, Soper D. *Infectious Diseases in Women.* New York, NY: McGraw-Hill; 2002.

Mandell G, Bennett J, Dolin R. *Principles and Practice of Infectious Diseases.* 6th ed New York, NY: Churchill Livingstone; 2006.

Moniff G, Baker D. *Infectious Diseases in Obstetrics and Gynecology.* 5th ed. Nashville, TN: Parthenon Publishing; 2004.

Postpartum Depression

THE PATIENT ENCOUNTER

You are seeing a 19-year-old woman (G1P1001) in your office for a postpartum visit. You notice that the young woman looks somewhat disheveled and you remember that she had always looked well-dressed and groomed at her prenatal visits. When asked about bonding with the baby, the patient becomes tearful and states, "I don't know if I can handle this."

OVERVIEW

Definition

Postpartum depression is defined as intense feelings of sadness, anxiety, or despair within 3 to 6 months following childbirth that interfere with the mother's ability to function. This should be differentiated from the "baby blues," which is a period of mild depressive mood and emotional lability that is self-limited (1). *Postpartum psychosis* is a very serious condition defined as lucidity that alternates with psychosis, confusion, and delirium during the postpartum period (2). This chapter will focus on the diagnosis and management of postpartum depression, as well as differentiating it from postpartum psychosis and the baby blues.

CLINICAL PEARL

According to the Diagnostic and Statistical Manual IV definitions, postpartum depression is really a major depressive disorder that happens within 4 weeks of delivery. The symptoms must be present almost every day for at least 2 weeks such that it begins to affect your ability to function at work, home, or in relationships.

Pathophysiology

The exact pathophysiology is unknown but many speculate that postpartum mood disorders are precipitated by the withdrawal of gonadotrophic hormones postpartum.

Epidemiology

Postpartum depression is a common problem and is estimated to affect 8 to 15% of women. The rate increases to 30% in adolescents and in women with a history of depressive illness. Seventy percent of women with a history of postpartum depression after a previous pregnancy will have subsequent postpartum depression; this increases to 85% if the woman currently has the baby blues (2). The baby blues may affect up to 50% of postpartum women. This condition begins 3 to 6 days postpartum and may continue for up 2 weeks. It resolves spontaneously and can be a normal part of the postpartum experience (1).

Postpartum psychosis occurs in 1 to 4 of 1,000 postpartum patients. In 25% of patients with postpartum psychosis, it will reoccur in the next pregnancy. Postpartum psychosis is usually a manifestation of an undiagnosed mood disorder. Women with bipolar disorder need to be carefully monitored for signs of psychosis. A woman is a greater risk for psychosis in the postpartum period than at any other time of her life (3). Risk factors for postpartum depression and postpartum psychosis are listed in Table 10-1.

Etiology

Postpartum depression and postpartum psychosis may be a manifestation of a previously undiagnosed mood disorder. Postpartum psychosis is associated with a personal or strong family history of bipolar disorder; any patient with a personal history of bipolar disorder needs to be observed for postpartum psychosis (3).

TABLE 10-1
Risk Factors Associated with Postpartum Depression and Psychosis

Postpartum Depression	Postpartum Psychosis
• Adolescence • History of depressive illness • History of postpartum depression • History of postpartum depression with the baby blues currently • Recent life stressors • Child care stress • Low self-esteem • Low socioeconomic status	• History of depression or severe life event in the past year • Young age • Primiparity • Family history of psychiatric disorders • History of bipolar disorder

Always remember that other physiological disorders can masquerade as mood disorders. Hypothyroidism, electrolyte imbalances, medications, drugs of abuse and, less commonly, brain lesions can also cause changes in mood and personality (3).

CLINICAL PEARL

The strongest predictor of postpartum depression is a maternal history of depression. In addition, women who have previously had postpartum depression are at an even higher risk of having a recurrent episode.

ACUTE MANAGEMENT AND WORKUP

Because postpartum depression is so common, the American College of Obstetricians and Gynecologists recommends briefly screening all postpartum women at their routine clinic visits.

The First 15 Minutes

Ask all patients two screening questions:

1. Over the past 2 weeks have you felt depressed, sad, or hopeless?
2. Over the past 2 weeks, have you lost interest or pleasure in your activities?

A positive response to both questions requires further assessment (1).

Initial Assessment

In evaluating a patient for postpartum depression, it is important to differentiate postpartum depression from the baby blues and also from postpartum psychosis.

Evaluation for Depression

Remember the signs of depression and ask specifically about each one. In a patient with depressed mood or anhedonia, four of the following criteria during the past 2 weeks qualify the patient as having a depressive episode:

1. *Sleep.* Patients with a major depressive disorder most often have insomnia and, less commonly, hypersomnia. Differentiate this from being kept awake by a crying baby or sleeping more during the day because the baby is awake all night.
2. *Interest.* A loss of interest or pleasure in usually enjoyable activities is almost always present in depression.
3. *Guilt.* A sense of worthlessness or guilt over situations that are not under the patient's control can be associated with depression.

4. *Energy*. Patients may complain of fatigue or loss of energy. Normal activities may exhaust them and take a longer amount of time.
5. *Concentration*. The patient may complain of being easily distracted or of having memory difficulties that affect her productivity.
6. *Appetite*. Appetite is usually decreased and patients may say they have to force themselves to eat. Occasionally, appetite may be increased with cravings for specific foods. This can cause significant weight loss or gain if continued for a long enough period of time.
7. *Psychomotor Changes*. Agitation or slowing may be observed by other people around the patient.
8. *Suicidal Thoughts*. Patients may have obsessive thoughts of death, suicidal ideation, or thoughts of harming the newborn baby. Obsessive thoughts need to be differentiated from delusions; obsessive thoughts are recognized as coming from the patient's mind, whereas delusional thoughts are perceived as coming from an outside source. You cannot predict which patient will harm herself or her baby; these patients need prompt psychiatric evaluation (4).

Evaluation for Psychosis

Also evaluate patients for signs of psychosis. Postpartum psychosis is a psychiatric emergency. Having one of the following qualifies the patient as having a psychotic episode:

1. *Delusions*. These can range from the patient thinking the baby is dead, that she or the baby is being persecuted, that the baby is possessed, and so on. Watch for delusions that involve the patient harming herself or the baby.
2. *Hallucinations*. These can be auditory, visual, olfactory, or gustatory. Specific attention must be paid to hallucinations that command the patient to harm herself or her baby.
3. *Disorganized Speech*. The patient's speech may be tangential and she does not make normal associations.
4. *Disorganized or Catatonic Behavior*. The patient often cannot perform necessary activities of daily living for herself or for the baby, which puts the child at risk from neglect (4).

Admission Criteria and Level of Care Criteria

The next step is to determine the patient's condition in the office.

Option 1: Stable Condition

When further questioned about her feelings, the patient states that she is very happy to have a new baby, although being a new mother is difficult. She states that she has mood swings and that when she is feeling sad, it usually only lasts for a few hours. Her husband states that her mood is unpredictable, that she can be happy one minute and crying the next. She states that she is able to continue to care for her baby and perform other activities of daily living without difficulty. Her social support system is strong and intact.

Option 2: Fair Condition
When further questioned about her feelings, the patient states that she is happy to have a new baby but feels very overwhelmed. She states that she feels like she cannot function and has difficulty completing daily tasks. She feels constantly sad and anxious and is worried that she will be a bad mother. Her husband states that she has seemed very sad and torpid, and that she will not get out of bed. She is worried because she has thoughts and fears of something bad happening to the baby.

Option 3: Critical Condition
When further questioned about her feelings, the patient states that the devil is trying to harm herself and her baby. Her husband is worried—he states that her mood is very erratic and she does not sleep much. He states that he has caught her talking to people who are not there and she has told him she needs to save the baby from the devil.

The First Few Hours

In a patient who is showing symptoms of postpartum psychosis or signs of postpartum depression with suicidal or homicidal ideations, urgent evaluation by a psychiatrist is needed. This will usually require admission to the hospital unless a psychiatrist is immediately available on an outpatient basis.

History

It is important to establish if the patient has a history of a previous psychiatric disorder. If she does have a psychiatric history, ask about previous treatment and hospitalization. Ask which medications she has taken in the past, including which have helped her, which did not, and if she had an adverse reaction to any medication. Take a family history to evaluate if any other members of her family have psychiatric disorders. Make sure to ask the patient about medications, alcohol use, and the use of illicit substances. Take a full review of systems.

The patient should be asked about suicidal or homicidal ideation. If the patient endorses either, she should be asked if she has a plan. Evaluate for hallucinations or delirium. Delusional altruistic homicide is a feature of postpartum psychosis in which the mother kills the infant and often then commits suicide to save the baby from the delusional perpetrator. Of people who commit infanticide, 40% had seen a health care provider prior to the incident (3). One study found that 5% of patients with postpartum psychosis committed suicide and 4% committed infanticide (5).

Physical Examination
The patient should be evaluated for signs of self-injury or of physical abuse. Evaluate the patient for a goiter or for neurologic deficits.

Labs and Tests to Consider
A thyrotropin and chemistry panel should be performed to evaluate for organic causes of depression. Other labs should be ordered based on the physical exam findings.

Imaging
Routine imaging is not required; however, if the patient has a neurologic deficit, imaging should be considered with the recommendation of a neurologist.

Treatment
After determining your patient's condition, the next step is to make a plan for management as outlined in Table 10-2 (2,3).

The Baby Blues
Treatment should be supportive. Reassure the patient and her family that the baby blues are transient and self-limited. Advise the patient and her family to be aware of signs of depression or psychosis.

Postpartum Depression
Treatment should be supportive and usually requires antidepressant medication. Postpartum depression should be managed in cooperation with a psychiatrist. The duration of depression is determined by the delay in receiving treatment. Observe the patient carefully for suicidal or homicidal ideation or for signs of psychosis.

Selective serotonin reuptake inhibitors are the first-line treatment for postpartum depression. Studies of fluoxetine, sertraline, venlafaxine, and fluvoxamine show efficacy at the same doses as those recommended for the general population. Tricyclic antidepressants have also been found to be as efficacious. In women who are breast-feeding, the exposure of the infant to antidepressant medications is much less than the exposure of the fetus. Sertraline, paroxetine, and nortriptyline are first-line medications in breast-feeding mothers because they do not produce quantifiable levels of drug or metabolite in the infant (3,5).

Postpartum Psychosis
Treatment should include urgent psychiatric consultation and usually hospitalization. Medications should be managed in close cooperation with a psychiatrist. Observe the patient for signs of suicidal or homicidal ideation. The

TABLE 10-2
Treatment of Postpartum Mood Disorders

Mood Disorder	Treatment	Medication	Warning Signs
Baby blues	Self-limited disorder; provide supportive care	None needed	If condition does not improve within 2 weeks, consider postpartum depression
Postpartum depression	Length of disease related to delay of treatment; supportive care with psychiatry	Not breast-feeding: first line, SSRI; second line, TCA. Breast-feeding: sertraline, paroxetine, and nortriptyline are first line	Patient needs close follow-up; coordinate with psychiatry. Watch for suicidal or homicidal ideations. Watch for evidence of psychosis
Postpartum psychosis	Needs urgent psychiatric treatment	May need a combination of antidepressants and antipsychotics; needs management by psychiatry	Watch for recurrence of hallucinations or delusions. Watch for potential for infanticide/suicide Watch for other mood disorders

SSRI, selective serotonin reuptake inhibitor; TCA, tricyclic antidepressant.

baby should be removed from the mother's care. If deemed appropriate, supervised visits with the baby are beneficial to the patient. If the patient is evaluated and decided that hospitalization is not warranted, the patient needs someone to assure she is caring for herself and is kept out of high-risk situations.

EXTENDED IN-HOSPITAL MANAGEMENT

The patient should be monitored in-house until she no longer has suicidal or homicidal ideation, or delusions or hallucinations. Management with psychiatric services is essential. Medication should be adjusted during this time and the patient should be observed for adverse reactions.

DISPOSITION

Discharge Goals

Prior to discharge from the hospital and directed observation by a physician, the patient must meet the following goals:

- The patient denies suicidal or homicidal ideation and is not having delusions or hallucinations.
- She can obtain her medications, can arrange for appropriate follow-up with psychiatric services, and is reliable enough to take her medications and come for her appointments.
- She has a support system at home.

Outpatient Care

For the baby blues, the patient can continue with routine postpartum clinic visits but she and her family should be aware of the signs of depression. Patients with postpartum depression or those recovering from postpartum psychosis need frequent visits to evaluate for signs of worsening condition or relapse. These patients need to have a psychiatrist involved in their care who can help to properly adjust their medications.

 WHAT YOU NEED TO REMEMBER

- The baby blues are a normal process and are self-limited, but women with this disorder are at higher risk for postpartum depression.
- Postpartum depression commonly affects women, and all postpartum women should be screened at clinic visits.
- Postpartum depression and psychosis should be treated in conjunction with a psychiatrist.

- Women with postpartum depression need to be carefully monitored for suicidal or homicidal ideation.
- Selective serotonin reuptake inhibitors are the first-line treatment for postpartum depression; remember to ask the patient if she is breast-feeding as this affects your medication choice.
- The duration of a postpartum depressive episode is determined by the delay to treatment.
- Postpartum psychosis is a psychiatric emergency and is rarely but tragically associated with suicide and infanticide.

REFERENCES

1. American College of Obstetricians and Gynecologists. ACOG committee opinion number 343: psychosocial risk factors: perinatal screening and intervention. *Obstet Gynecol.* 2006;108:469–477.
2. Cunningham FG, Leveno KJ, Bloom SL, et al. *Williams Obstetrics.* 22nd ed. New York, NY: McGraw-Hill; 2005.
3. Gabbe SG, Niebyl JR, Simpson JL. *Obstetrics: Normal and Problem Pregnancies.* 5th ed. New York, NY: Churchill Livingstone; 2007.
4. First BM. *Diagnostic and Statistical Manual of Mental Disorders: DSM-IV-TR.* 4th ed. Arlington, VA: American Psychiatric Association; 2000.
5. Sadock BJ, Sadock VA. *Kaplan and Sadock's Synopsis of Psychiatry.* 9th ed. Philadelphia, PA: Lippincott Williams & Wilkins; 2000.

THE PATIENT ENCOUNTER

An 18-year-old woman (G0) presents to your office 48 hours after having unprotected intercourse. She is in a monogamous relationship with her boyfriend and they are both freshmen at the local university. There is no history of sexually transmitted diseases and she has only been sexually active with one partner. She does not want to be pregnant and wants to know what her options are.

OVERVIEW

Definition

Contraception is a strategy used to prevent unintended pregnancies. Contraception can be either permanent or reversible, and it can be hormonal or nonhormonal. There are many reasons for seeking contraception. Whether to space children; to postpone childbearing for a career, a relationship, or financial reasons, or to prevent pregnancy due to pre-exiting diseases such as severe aortic stenosis, Eisenmenger syndrome, or numerous other reasons, physicians must be prepared to instruct patients and prescribe appropriate contraception for all their patients' needs.

Pathophysiology

In the case of reversible contraception, there are two basic classes of contraception: hormonal and nonhormonal methods. Hormonal methods have a progestin component and with or without estrogen component. The progestin component is what primarily offers contraceptive efficacy through its ability to inhibit ovulation, thicken cervical mucus, slow down the motility of cilia found in the fallopian tubes, and alter the glycogen production of the endometrium. In contraception in which a synthetic estrogen is included (like the oral contraceptive pill), the estrogen component helps to prevent unwanted, unscheduled uterine bleeding, and is thought to hinder follicular development. Emergency contraception is believed to work by inhibiting ovulation with a high dose of progestins.

There are a number of nonhormonal methods of contraception, each with a slightly different mechanism of action. The barrier methods act to physically prevent the fertilization of an egg with sperm. Spermicides, such as nonoxynol 9, act by killing sperm on contact by destroying the sperm's cell membrane. Finally, natural family planning uses a variety of techniques to predict your patient's most fertile days of the month. This information is used to help couples decide when to abstain from having unprotected intercourse (1).

Epidemiology

In the United States, there are approximately 62 million women of reproductive age (between 15 and 44 years of age). Of the 62 million women, approximately two thirds of them are currently using one form of contraception, and more than 95% of those who have ever had sex have used at least one method of contraception in the past.

Of those women who are actively using contraception, two-thirds use a reversible method, such as condoms or oral contraceptive pills (OCPs). In women younger than age 30, the OCP is the leading method of contraception; women older than age 35 tend to rely on sterilization. Finally, when comparing age-matched populations, African American and Hispanic women primarily use sterilization for contraception whereas white women primarily use an OCP (2).

CLINICAL PEARL

Worldwide, intrauterine devices (IUDs) are the most common form of reversible contraception used.

Etiology

Contraception is not a new concept; throughout history many methods have been tried. Coitus interruptus was widely used and referred to in works by Ebers Papyrus that date back to 1550 BC. Condoms as a method to prevent venereal disease were described by Fallopius in the early 16th century. By the mid-20th century, the first reports of success with an oral contraceptive pill for women were produced (3).

ACUTE MANAGEMENT AND WORKUP

Time is of the essence when working with a patient who is in need of emergency contraception. Success rates exponentially decrease 72 hours after unprotected coitus, but should be made available to women who request it up to 120 hours.

The First 15 Minutes

Establishing a relationship with the patient that promotes an uninhibited conversation and trust is key to the successful management of a patient in emergent need of contraception. The discussion should be nonjudgmental and educational, using open-ended questions.

Initial Assessment

Obtain a complete history, paying particular attention to the patient's past gynecologic history. A detailed menstrual history, including the date of last period and the regularity of menses, is critical for counseling the patient about the likelihood of ovulation. A detailed contraceptive and sexual history will play a role in the long-term contraceptive management plan.

Admission Criteria and Level of Care Criteria

In the absence of a known pregnancy undergoing an active miscarriage, admission for emergency contraception is not indicated.

The First Few Hours

Once a trusting doctor-patient relationship has been established, the provider can focus on the counseling aspect of emergency contraception.

History

When you are performing a well-woman examination on someone of reproductive age (ages 15 to 44), you should always ask about their obstetric history and desires for future fertility. This will give you an opportunity to discuss emergency contraception and ways to prevent getting a sexually transmitted disease. Finally, a detailed medical history is important to document as you begin to look for contraindications to certain forms of contraception (such as the OCP).

Physical Examination

A general gynecologic exam is not unreasonable prior to initiating contraception. If the patient's history does not make sense or there are other physical signs suggestive of abuse or an alleged criminal assault, a detailed physical exam, including a full-body survey for bruises or lacerations, is mandatory.

Labs and Tests to Consider

While performing the pelvic exam, a wet prep along with cultures for gonorrhea and chlamydia are standard in women who are sexually active and 25 years of age or younger. If the patient has high-risk sexual practices, testing for other sexually transmitted diseases, including human immunodeficiency virus, hepatitis B, and syphilis, is reasonable. This is also a prime opportunity to ensure that the patient is current with her Pap smear.

Key Diagnostic Labs and Tests

Although not necessary prior to the initiation of emergency contraception, a urine pregnancy test is recommended if the patient is available to provide a urine specimen. If the urine pregnancy test is positive, then a serum beta-human chorionic gonadotropin is necessary to further evaluate the pregnancy and its location.

Imaging

In the presence of a positive urine pregnancy test, a transvaginal ultrasound should be performed to assess for a uterine or nonuterine pregnancy. An ectopic pregnancy is a gynecologic emergency and confers a significant risk of morbidity if the diagnosis is missed.

Treatment

The failure rate of emergency contraception is 2% using oral contraceptives and 1% with levonorgestrel. Levonorgestrel (Plan B) is the treatment of choice because it has fewer side effects (nausea and vomiting) and greater efficacy. Some practitioners suggest prescribing emergency contraception to those who choose barrier contraceptives because of the risk of failure of barrier contraceptives as well as the need to be able to access emergency contraception without difficulty if failure occurs. Treatment options for emergency contraception include the following:

- Levonorgestrel (Plan B)—Administer 750 mcg by mouth within 120 hours and repeat in 12 hours (no estrogen component = fewer side effects)
- Yuzpe method—Uses OCPs as emergency contraception. Listed here are some brands and their dosing (the American College of Obstetricians and Gynecologists has a complete listing available in Practice Bulletin 69).
  - Ovral: two tablets followed by two tablets 12 hours later
  - Alesse: five tablets followed by five tablets 12 hours later
  - Lo/Ovral, Nordette, Levlen, Triphasil, Tri-Levlen: four tablets followed by four tablets 12 hours later
- Copper IUD—Effective within 120 hours of unprotected intercourse

> **CLINICAL PEARL**
>
> *Success rates exponentially decrease 72 hours after unprotected coitus, but should be made available to women who request it up to 120 hours. Emergency contraception should be initiated as soon as possible after unprotected intercourse or inadequately protected intercourse.*

EXTENDED MANAGEMENT

In addition to providing emergency contraception in a timely manner, helping the patient establish an acceptable and reliable long-term contraceptive plan is essential for any patient desiring to reduce the chances of getting pregnant.

Methods of Contraception

When you are discussing contraception with your patient, knowing all of the different options and their relative contraindications will allow you and your patient to choose a method that will be acceptable to her and that will ensure a high compliance rate. If you ask your patient the following two simple questions, it will significantly tailor your choice for contraception: (a) *Do you prefer pills or no pills?* and (b) *Can you remember to use something daily or would you prefer a longer dosing schedule?*

Traditional, Nonhormonal Methods of Contraception

The primary methods of traditional, nonhormonal contraception include coitus interruptus, lactational amenorrhea, and periodic abstinence.

- Lactational Amenorrhea—If a mother is using breast-feeding as the infant's primary source of nutrition, lactational amenorrhea is a safe contraceptive method to use for up to 6 months. After that time, another method becomes necessary; when menses resumes, another contraceptive method will be needed.
- Periodic Abstinence—This method involves the calendar or rhythm method, the cervical mucus method, and the symptothermal (or temperature) method. Failure rate is approximately 20%.

Also known as natural family planning, periodic abstinence focuses on establishing a woman's fertile period and avoiding intercourse during this time. Known facts concerning this timing include the sperm's ability to survive in the female reproductive tract (2 to 7 days) and the lifespan of the ovum (1 to 3) days.

There are three methods for calculating the woman's most fertile period of time: (a) calendar or rhythm method (Fig. 11-1), (b) cervical mucous method, and (c) symptothermal method. Of the three techniques, the symptothermal method is the most accurate. It uses a record of basal body temperature along with cervical mucus to predict ovulation. Nevertheless, the establishment of regular cycles is essential for this technique to work.

Spermicides

Spermicides do not protect against sexually transmitted infections. The primary spermicides include vaginal contraceptive film, foams, jellies and creams, and vaginal suppositories. Failure rates range between 20 and 50%.

Barrier Methods of Contraception

The main types of barrier methods include condoms (for both males and females) (Fig. 11-2), the cervical cap, the diaphragm, and the contraceptive

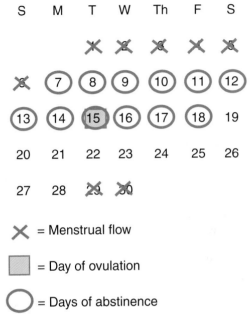

FIGURE 11-1: Calendar method of natural family planning.

sponge. One of the main advantages of barrier methods of contraception is the significant reduction in the transmission rate of both viral and bacterial sexually transmitted infections. The disadvantage is the need to plan ahead in order to apply the barrier before intercourse. Failure rates of male condoms are approximately 11%.

Oral Contraception

The estrogen component of most OCPs is ethinyl estradiol. The progestin component of OCPs has evolved over time. Pills are often selected based on its progestin component. Several forms are available:

- Desogestrel, norgestimate, and gestodene are newer progestins that all have reduced androgenicity (acne and hirsutism) while maintaining cycle control.
- Drospirenone (spironolactone analogue) has both antiandrogenic and antimineralocorticoid activity. It decreases water retention and appetite.

OCPs come in either monophasic preparations (a constant amount of estrogen and progesterone) or a multiphasic preparation (varying doses of

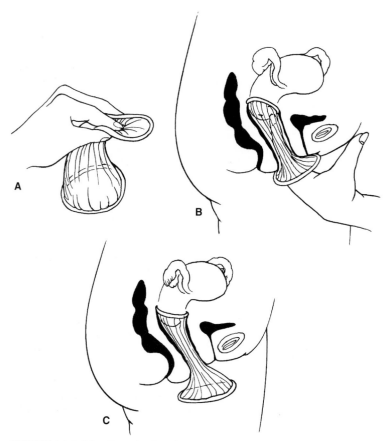

FIGURE 11-2: **The Female Condom**. Preparation for insertion (**A**), insertion (**B**), and condom in proper position (**C**).

either estrogen and/or progesterone). Combination OCPs do have associated risks when used in women with coexisting medical conditions, particularly those that predispose to developing thrombosis. Some absolute contraindications to the use of OCPs include the following (4):

- Thrombophlebitis, thromboembolic disorders (including personal or close family history, such as parent or sibling), cerebral vascular disease, coronary occlusion, or conditions predisposing to these conditions
- Known or suspected breast cancer
- Undiagnosed abnormal vaginal bleeding
- Known or suspected pregnancy

- Smokers older than age 35
- Elevated blood pressure or uncontrolled hypertension
- Migraines with aura (classic)

Despite the risks associated with the use of OCPs, there are numerous noncontraceptive benefits your patients should be aware of. These include:

- Reductions in dysmenorrhea
- Reductions in endometriosis-related symptoms
- Treatment of acne and hirsutism
- Prevention of functional ovarian cysts
- Improvement in premenstrual syndrome symptoms
- Increased bone density
- Decreased incidence of endometrial and ovarian cancer
- Fewer ectopic pregnancies
- Possible decrease in the incidence of benign breast disease and rheumatoid arthritis

You have to carefully weigh your patient's individual risks and benefits before prescribing OCPs. Failure rates for combined OCPs is between 1% and 2% and approximately 2% for progestin-only pills.

Progestin-Only Contraception

Progestin-only contraception allows physicians to find efficacious contraception while eliminating the estrogen-related risks. Examples of this form of birth control are progestin-only OCPs (Micronor), medroxyprogesterone acetate in depot form (injectable), Implanon, and the levonorgestrel IUD system (Mirena). The main disadvantage of this form of contraception is the high frequency of abnormal bleeding patterns and the resulting reduced patient compliance.

Injectable Contraception

Depot-medroxyprogesterone acetate was approved for contraception in the United States in 1992, but it has been used in many countries since the mid-1960s. This progestin-only contraception inhibits ovulation and thickens cervical mucus. The dose is 150 mg intramuscularly or 104 mg subcutaneously every 3 months, and it is an excellent choice for those who have trouble with compliance. It is also a useful choice in situations in which there is a need for improved hygiene in patients not able to care for themselves. Because there is no estrogen component, depot-medroxyprogesterone acetate is used commonly for those with congenital heart disease, sickle cell anemia, a prior history of thromboembolism, as well as for patients with seizure disorders or women older than age 30 who smoke or have other risk factors. Its major side effect is irregular bleeding (70% incidence in first year of use); others include weight gain (2 to 5 pounds over the first year of use), bone loss, which is reversible after discontinuation, and depression. However, after 1 year of treatment, 55% of patients experience amenorrhea. Failure rates are <1%.

Transdermal Contraception

The NuvaRing is a vaginal, transparent ring that administers 15 mcg of ethinyl estradiol and 120 mcg of etonogestrel. The vaginal route avoids gastrointestinal absorption and first-pass liver effect. The ring is inserted by the patient and is worn for 3 weeks; it is then removed and left out for a week, and a new ring is placed. The circulating progestin and estrogen are only 40% and 30%, respectively, of the corresponding levels with OCPs.

The transdermal contraceptive patch (Ortho Evra) is similar in that one patch (20 cm^2) is worn for 1 week for 3 consecutive weeks; the patch is then removed and left off for a week and a new kit is begun. The patch delivers 20 mcg of ethinyl estradiol and 150 mcg of norelgestromin each day. Application should be to the lower abdomen, the upper outer arm, or the buttock or upper torso (excluding the breast). Detachment occurs 5% of the time and usually with inexperienced patients. Failure rates are similar to OCPs. The main disadvantage of both transdermal methods of contraception is remembering when to change the device (i.e., weekly versus monthly).

Implantable Contraception

Implanon offers long-term, reversible, progestin-only contraception via an implantable rod in the upper arm. The 4-cm rod contains etonogestrel, released at a daily rate that decreases by half after 2 years. This method of contraception lasts 3 years. The Implanon is easily inserted and removed in your office. Its predecessor, Norplant, was a similar system, using five implantable rods. Norplant is no longer sold in the United States.

Intrauterine Devices

The mechanism of action is not well understood, but the current belief is that a hostile environment is created by mobilizing leukocytes as a foreign body reaction. These devices can easily be inserted in your office (Fig. 11-3). In addition, they have a monofilament string attached that passes through the cervical canal and that can be grasped for removal during a pelvic exam. Two common noteworthy points are that IUDs are *not* abortifacients and IUDs *do not* increase the risk of ectopic pregnancy.

The two IUDs marketed in the United States are the Mirena, which contains progesterone (20 mcg/d levonorgestrel), and the ParaGard (T 380A), the only nonhormonal, copper-bearing IUD marketed in the United States.

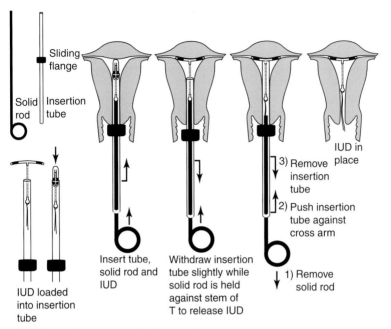

Sliding flange

Solid rod

Insertion tube

3) Remove insertion tube

2) Push insertion tube against cross arm

1) Remove solid rod

IUD in place

Insert tube, solid rod and IUD

Withdraw insertion tube slightly while solid rod is held against stem of T to release IUD

IUD loaded into insertion tube

FIGURE 11-3: Insertion of a ParaGard intrauterine device.

> **CLINICAL PEARL**
>
> *The Mirena must be replaced every 5 years, whereas the ParaGard is good for 10 years.*

Absolute contraindications to IUD use are the following:

- Undiagnosed vaginal bleeding
- Acute infection
- Current pregnancy
- Past history of salpingitis
- Suspected gynecologic malignancy

Sterilization

Permanent sterilization is accomplished by four methods: (a) insertion of a nickel coil, (b) tubal ligation, (c) laparoscopic tubal sterilization, and (d) vasectomy. Details related to sterilization are discussed in Chapter 12.

DISPOSITION

Discharge Goals

After a patient initiates contraception, it is important to emphasize the need for backup contraception until efficacy is established. In addition, patients may notice a brief period of abnormal menses in the case of hormonal contraception. Counseling should always include a discussion of safe sex habits and a reminder that sexually transmitted diseases are prevented only using barrier contraception.

Outpatient Care

When a patient initiates a new form of contraception, it is recommended that she have a follow-up visit in 1 month. This visit allows the patient an opportunity to ask you any questions she has regarding her new form of contraception. In addition, any potential compliance issues can be addressed and corrected.

 WHAT YOU NEED TO REMEMBER

- Know and counsel patients regarding the risks, benefits, and contraindications of oral contraceptives.
- The progestin component of OCPs provides the main contraception benefit. The estrogen component of OCPs helps to minimize the amount of abnormal uterine bleeding.
- IUDs are best placed during or just after menstrual cycles as the cervical canal is patent.
- Emergency contraception should be offered/made available to women who have had unprotected intercourse or inadequately protected intercourse who do not desire pregnancy.
- Levonorgestrel-only regimen (Plan B) is more effective for emergency contraception and has fewer side effects, and should be the first-line agent.
- The copper IUD may be used for emergency contraception up to 120 hours (5 days) after unprotected intercourse.

REFERENCES

1. Katz. Family planning: contraception, sterilization, and pregnancy termination. In: Mishell D, Jr. *Comprehensive Gynecology.* 5th ed. St. Louis, MO: CV Mosby; 2007.
2. Mosher WD, Martinez GM, Chandra A, et al. Use of contraception and use of family planning services in the United States: 1982–2002, Advance Data from Vital and Health Statistics, No. 350. Hyattsville, MD: National Center for Health Statistics, 2004.

3. Fraser IS. Forty years of combined oral contraception: the evolution of a revolution. *Med J Aust.* 2000;173(10):541–544.
4. American College of Obstetricians and Gynecologists. ACOG practice bulletin number 69:emergency contraception. *Obstet Gynecol.* 2005;106:1443–1452.

SUGGESTED READINGS

American College of Obstetricians and Gynecologists. ACOG practice bulletin number 73: use of hormonal contraception in women with coexisting medical conditions. *Obstet Gynecol.* 2006:107:1453–1472.
American College of Obstetricians and Gynecologists. ACOG committee opinion number 337: noncontraceptive uses of the levonorgestrel intrauterine system. *Obstet Gynecol.* 2006;107:1479–1482.

Sterilization

THE PATIENT ENCOUNTER

At morning rounds, your postpartum patient requests information about her options for birth control. She is a 31-year-old woman (G4P4) who had a routine vaginal delivery of a healthy child, and she is being discharged from the hospital today. She plans to breast-feed her baby and states that she is not interested in taking pills for contraception. She now has four healthy children, is in a successful marriage, and says her family "is complete."

OVERVIEW

Definition

Sterilization in the form of a surgical procedure is a highly effective and permanent means of contraception. The rate of surgical sterilization in both men and women has increased over the past several years and it is important to appreciate the various types of procedures available to patients. You should also understand the counseling process that is involved in a patient's decision to proceed with a permanent sterilization procedure.

Pathophysiology

Permanent sterilization is achieved by either mechanical interruption or removal of part of the fallopian tubes or vas deferens. The goal is to prevent sperm from fertilizing the egg. It is important to appreciate that despite being referred to as "permanent" sterilization, there is a well-documented risk of failure.

Epidemiology

It is estimated that approximately 25% of reproductive age women will choose sterilization as their method of contraception each year. Of those, approximately 70% are female sterilization methods and 25% are vasectomies (1). The rate of sterilization procedures is higher in women who are older than age 30, are currently married, and are African American. It is currently considered the most common method of contraception.

ACUTE MANAGEMENT AND WORKUP

Sterilization is not a procedure that should be performed in the acute setting without a previously well-documented counseling session between you and your patient.

The First Few Hours

For patients who desire a form of permanent sterilization, appropriate counseling should be provided, with informed consent being obtained for the procedure. Patients should be given all the options that are available for contraception. The patient must also express a desire for no further childbearing. Once a decision is made for sterilization, the patient should be given information regarding the various procedure types, the risks associated with an operation, the failure rates, and possible complications.

History

A detailed medical history should be obtained from the patient prior to the procedure. It is important to establish any medical diagnoses that prohibit the use of hormone contraceptives or place the patient at risk for a complicated pregnancy. This information can help to guide the physician in his or her management of a patient with undesired fertility by offering permanent sterilization.

Pertinent medical conditions that meet these criteria include but are not limited to:

- A history of thromboembolic disease (e.g., deep vein thrombosis, pulmonary thromboembolism) or coagulopathy
- A history of a cerebral vascular accident or ischemic heart disease
- A history of an estrogen-dependent tumor or a history of breast cancer
- Patient age >35 with current tobacco use
- Migraines with focal neurologic symptoms
- Uncontrolled hypertension or diabetes
- Liver disease
- Chronic heart disease

Physical Examination

A routine physical exam should be performed preoperatively on any patient undergoing a surgical procedure. A detailed surgical history should be obtained from the patient prior to the procedure. It is important to establish any risk factors or concerns that may influence the route of the surgical procedure. Knowledge of prior abdominal surgeries is critical to making this decision. A patient with prior complications from anesthesia may also influence the choice of route of sterilization.

Labs and Tests to Consider

Because the sterilization procedure is deemed to carry minimal operative risk, the only lab tests necessary to perform are those dictated by the patient's past medical history. It is important to have a urine pregnancy test on the day of the procedure. In addition, it is useful to document when the patient's last menstrual period was and what form of contraception the patient had been using prior to the surgical procedure.

Treatment

There are two general classes of tubal sterilization procedures that are based on when the procedure is performed: postpartum and interval procedures. If a patient is stable following delivery by vaginal route, the decision to proceed with a *postpartum* tubal ligation can occur immediately. Tubal sterilization can also occur at the time of cesarean section. Usually these procedures are discussed with the patient prior to delivery. If a patient presents at a time not associated with pregnancy, an *interval* sterilization procedure can be scheduled.

Counseling

A discussion of contraceptive options should be completed with the patient prior to obtaining informed consent. The patient must understand that sterilization is a permanent procedure. Other important factors that should be discussed include the following:

• The reason for choosing permanent sterilization
• Whether or not the patient is in a stable relationship or marriage (either of these will decrease postprocedure regret)
• The need for continued protection against sexually transmitted diseases through condom use
• That no change in menstrual flow should occur after the procedure
• An understanding of failure rates
• An understanding of the general risks and complications associated with surgery
• That sterilization provides a small degree of protection against ovarian cancer

A patient who desires a sterilization procedure must be informed of the failure rates that are commonly noted in the literature. These rates are based on information that is derived from the CREST study (Collaborative Review of Sterilization), which followed approximately 10,000 patients for 10 years following sterilization. From this study, the failure rate typically reported was 18.5 of 1,000 procedures (1.85%) when including all types. However, postpartum tubal ligations were noted to have a failure rate of only 7.5 per 1,000, the lowest of all types of procedures performed. The highest rates of failure were noted to occur with spring clip application and bipolar cautery (36 and 25 per 1,000 procedures, respectively). These data may influence the surgeon's decision to perform a particular procedure (2).

CLINICAL PEARL

It is important to realize that sterilization failures continue to happen years after the sterilization. Therefore, the cumulative 10-year failure rates are most helpful when counseling your patients. Each method has a different 10-year cumulative failure rate: 3.7% for spring clip, 2.5% for bipolar coagulation, 1.1% for vasectomies, and 0.8% for postpartum partial salpingectomy.

Female Sterilization

Once a patient has been prepared for surgery and informed consent has been obtained, the desired procedure can be performed. In the immediate postpartum period, a minilaparotomy incision is typically made beneath the umbilicus to visualize the fallopian tubes. The most common techniques involve grasping the tube and performing a partial salpingectomy (Fig. 12-1). This can also be done simultaneously with a cesarean section. Advantages of this route include the need for less technical expertise, the use of regional rather than general anesthesia, no increase in the length of the hospital stay, and retrieval of a pathologic specimen. Disadvantages

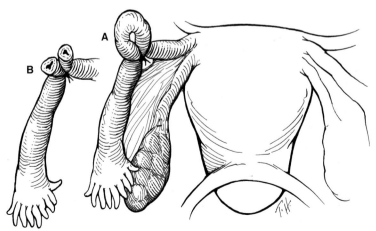

FIGURE 12-1: Pomeroy technique for tubal sterilization.

include a larger incision and an increased need for postpartum pain medications.

For a patient who desires sterilization that is not related to a current pregnancy, an interval procedure can be performed. Most procedures are performed via laparoscopy under general anesthesia. Techniques include mechanical occlusion of the tubes with clips/rings or ligation of the tubes by using electrocautery or sutures (Figs. 12-2 and 12-3). Advantages of this route include a decrease in operative time, less postoperative pain, and a rapid return to normal activity. Disadvantages include need for general anesthesia and a risk of intraoperative complications (such as bowel injury or hemorrhage).

An additional interval technique called Essure was introduced in 2002. This is a minimally invasive method of permanent sterilization that is performed via hysteroscopy. The Essure device (Conceptus, Mountain View, CA) is introduced through the hysteroscope (transcervically) and small coils are placed into the proximal aspect of each fallopian tube. The coils are designed to stimulate growth of the surrounding tissue around the coils, thereby occluding the tubes. The procedure can be done with local anesthesia and minimal sedation to the patient. Occlusion of the fallopian tubes occurs over

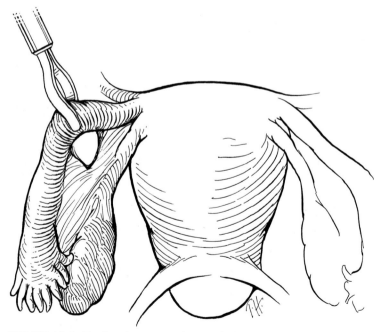

FIGURE 12-2: Bipolar electrocoagulation tubal sterilization.

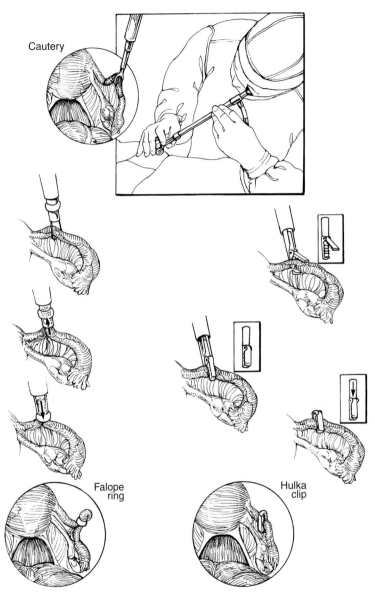

Cautery

Falope
ring

Hulka
clip

FIGURE 12-3: Laparoscopic sterilization.

a 3-month period, which must be proven with a hysterosalpingogram at that time. The procedure has been studied for 5 years and is currently reporting a 99.7% efficacy rate. Advantages include the ability to perform the procedure in the office, no incision, less cost to the patient, and its being an optimal therapy for patients with contraindications to surgery and/or anesthesia. The major disadvantage is the need for 3 months of contraception following the procedure and the necessity to perform a hysterosalpingogram to visualize tubal occlusion.

Male Sterilization

Another option for permanent sterilization is vasectomy for male patients. This procedure may be preferred to female sterilization because it is more cost-effective, requires only local anesthesia, and has an equal success rate in preventing future pregnancy. Complications following vasectomy are usually minor and are most commonly hematoma and incisional infection. Men do remain fertile for a period of time after the procedure and azoospermia must be confirmed by semen analysis. This is usually done 3 months after the procedure.

EXTENDED IN-HOSPITAL MANAGEMENT

These procedures are generally performed in an outpatient setting and rarely require in-hospital management. The only exception is when the female sterilization procedure is performed in conjunction with a vaginal delivery or cesarean delivery. The sterilization procedure is minor and in-hospital management would primarily focus on recovering from the obstetric event.

DISPOSITION

Discharge Goals

The rate of postoperative complication following sterilizations is about 1%. Postoperative complications are usually mild, such as hematoma or wound infection. The rate of major complications, such as the need for major surgery, bowel injury, or uterine perforation, is <1%. Complications resulting from anesthesia can also occur.

Outpatient Care

Pregnancy is rare following sterilization procedures, but failure rates should be discussed with the patient prior to the procedure using the statistics noted earlier. In addition, the risk of ectopic pregnancy is increased in comparison to the general population. Data from the CREST study estimate that the risk of ectopic pregnancy after sterilization is about 7.3 per 1,000 procedures (2). The risk is highest following bipolar cauterization.

WHAT YOU NEED TO REMEMBER

- Review all contraceptive options with the patient and obtain informed consent for the procedure. The patient must understand that the surgical procedure is permanent.
- The patient must understand that the procedure does not prevent transmission of sexually transmitted infections.
- The complications and side effects of tubal sterilization are minimal but should be reviewed prior to the procedure.
- Vasectomy is also an option that provides similar efficacy to that of female surgery with less risk of complications after procedure.
- Surgical sterilization is considered permanent.

REFERENCES

1. Katz VL, Lentz GM, Lobo RA, et al. *Comprehensive Gynecology.* 5th ed. Philadelphia, PA: Mosby Elsevier, 2007.
2. Peterson HB, Xia Z, Hughes JM, et al. The risk of pregnancy after tubal sterilization: findings from the U.S. Collaborative Review of Sterilization. *Am J Obstet Gynecol.* 1996;174:1161–1168.

SUGGESTED READINGS

American College of Obstetricians and Gynecologists. ACOG practice bulletin number 46, 2003: benefits and risks of sterilization. *Obstet Gynecol.* 2007;102:647–658.
American College of Obstetricians and Gynecologists. ACOG committee opinion number 371, 2007: sterilization of women, including those with mental disabilities. *Obstet Gynecol.* 2007;110:217–220.
American College of Obstetricians and Gynecologists. ACOG practice bulletin number 369: Multifetal pregnancy reduction. *Obstet Gynecol.* 2007;109:1511–1515.

13 Ectopic Pregnancy

THE PATIENT ENCOUNTER

A 19-year-old woman (G3P2) presents to the emergency department with right lower quadrant pain that began approximately 1 hour prior to arrival. She reports feeling short of breath and dizzy. Her past medical history is significant for a chlamydial infection treated 6 months ago. Her blood pressure is 90/60 mm Hg with a heart rate of 125 beats per minute. A positive pregnancy test is obtained.

OVERVIEW

Definition

An ectopic pregnancy is a pregnancy that implants in a location other then the endometrium (1). The fallopian tube is the most common location for an ectopic pregnancy to occur. Most fallopian tube pregnancies are located in the ampulla. Some less common sites to find ectopic pregnancies are the cervix, the ovary, the cornua, or the abdomen (Fig. 13-1).

Pathophysiology

Acute inflammation secondary to upper genital infections leads to tubal damage, which subsequently predisposes patients to ectopic pregnancies. Some clinicians hypothesize that persistent chlamydial antigens trigger a delayed hypersensitivity-type reaction that can further damage fallopian tubes despite negative genital cultures.

Epidemiology

Ectopic pregnancy is the leading cause of maternal death in the first trimester (2). The incidence of ectopic pregnancy is on the rise. The Centers for Disease Control and Prevention (3) reports 17,800 women were hospitalized for ectopic pregnancy in 1970 compared with 88,400 in 1989 and 108,800 in 1992. This perceived rise in incidence is explained by three facts. First, our ability to diagnose ectopic pregnancies has improved with advent of high-resolution transvaginal ultrasound (4). Second, scarring related to tubal surgery has significantly contributed to the increase in ectopic pregnancies (4). Finally, scarring secondary to pelvic inflammatory diseases inhibits the ability of a blastocyst to freely travel down the fallopian tube.

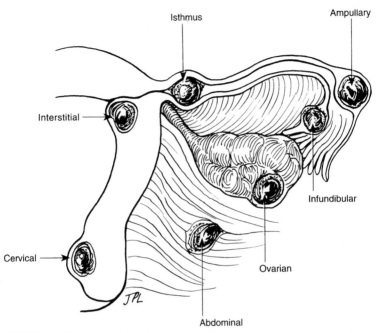

FIGURE 13-1: Potential locations of ectopic pregnancy.

CLINICAL PEARL

Ectopic pregnancies are the leading cause of maternal deaths in the first trimester of pregnancy because of hemorrhage.

Etiology

It normally takes an embryo formed in the fallopian tubes 7 gestational days to pass into the uterine cavity and implant (4). Anything that prevents the embryo from moving through the tube may result in implantation anywhere outside the endometrium.

The most common reason for delayed transport of an embryo is scarring secondary to pelvic infections. Incidentally, the most common culprit is *Chlamydia trachomatis*. Tubal surgery can also cause adhesions to form. These adhesions can be in the tube or external to the tube, which would prevent normal motility. Finally, there is some evidence that an imbalance of estrogen and progesterone can interfere with contractility of the fallopian tube.

Signs and Symptoms

The classic triad of symptoms for a patient with an ectopic pregnancy is abdominal pain, amenorrhea, and irregular vaginal bleeding (5). Patients may describe the pain as colicky, diffuse, or localized. The amount of pain is determined by the state of the ectopic pregnancy. Patients with unruptured ectopic pregnancies mostly complain of colicky pain secondary to tubal distention. Once an ectopic pregnancy ruptures, patients may complain of sharp, diffuse pain. This is due to irritation of the peritoneum as a result of bleeding from the ruptured ectopic pregnancy.

Differential Diagnosis

The differential diagnosis of ectopic pregnancy includes the following:

• Salpingitis
• Threatened or spontaneous abortion
• Appendicitis
• Ovarian torsion
• Hemorrhagic corpus luteum cyst

ACUTE MANAGEMENT AND WORKUP

Rapid recognition of an ectopic pregnancy is key to preventing what is known to be the leading cause of maternal mortality in the first trimester. If you follow the algorithm outlined later in this chapter (see Fig. 13-3), your evaluation of an ectopic pregnancy will efficiently confirm the diagnosis.

The First 15 Minutes

The most important question to answer in the first 15 minutes of an encounter with a patient who you suspect has an ectopic pregnancy is an assessment of her hemodynamic stability. Severe hemorrhage secondary to a ruptured ectopic pregnancy is a surgical emergency.

Initial Assessment

Recognizing an ectopic pregnancy is extremely important. The diagnosis of ectopic pregnancy is not always obvious, so you should proceed with a systematic approach. But before obtaining the history and performing the physical exam, the patient's initial appearance will alert you to the acuity of the disease.

Admission Criteria and Level of Care Criteria

If the patient is in severe pain and/or has signs and symptoms suggestive of hemorrhagic shock, admission is recommended. At this point, the patient should be approached as one would approach an emergent trauma patient.

The First Few Hours

After the patient has been stabilized hemodynamically by obtaining intravenous (IV) access with two large-bore IVs and inserting a Foley catheter to monitor for urine output, a thorough and systematic assessment should be performed.

History

You should obtain a focused history geared toward identifying risk factors that increase the likelihood of the patient having an ectopic pregnancy. To establish the patient's history, ask her the following questions:

- When did the pain begin?
- What is the quality of pain?
- When was your last menstrual period?
- Is there any history of previous ectopic pregnancy, sexually transmitted diseases, or tubal surgery?

Physical Examination

A careful abdominal/pelvic exam can help differentiate between a gastrointestinal and gynecologic process. First, you should focus on the abdominal exam. Look for any signs of rebound tenderness or guarding, which would suggest a surgical abdomen that requires immediate intervention. Next, perform a sterile speculum exam and look for any signs of a miscarriage, such as vaginal bleeding, a dilated cervix, or products of conception at the cervical os. Finally, you should perform a gentle bimanual exam, looking for any evidence of cervical motion tenderness or adnexal fullness/tenderness.

Labs and Tests to Consider

After you perform your exam, you should consider obtaining a few blood tests. You can look for evidence of acute blood loss anemia by getting a complete blood count. A blood type is important because women who are Rh-negative may need RhoGAM. Liver function tests and a serum creatinine are helpful if your patient is being evaluated for medical therapy using methotrexate.

Key Diagnostic Labs and Tests

In addition to the basic lab tests previously described, there are two main hormone levels that can provide useful information at the time of counseling. First, a serum beta-human chorionic gonadotropin (β-hCG) is the most important test to obtain. In normal pregnancies, the serum β-hCG rises in a log-linear fashion until around 70 days after the last menstrual period. When sampled 48 hours apart, the serum value should rise 53% to 66%. A difference <53% should alert you about a possible abnormal pregnancy of unknown location.

Next, a serum progesterone can offer information that would be useful while counseling your patient about the long-term prognosis of the pregnancy. A progesterone level <5 ng/mL is consistent with an abnormal pregnancy (not just an ectopic pregnancy). A progesterone level >20 ng/mL is consistent with a normal pregnancy (although ectopic pregnancies can occur with high progesterone levels). The key to remember is that progesterone levels do not identify location of pregnancies, just the likelihood of the pregnancy being normal.

CLINICAL PEARL

In early pregnancy, the serum β-hCG level should rise at least 53% every 48 hours in normal pregnancies. An abnormal rising pattern should alert you to suspect an abnormal pregnancy.

Imaging

The most important fact to confirm is whether the pregnancy is in the uterus or is extrauterine. Ultrasonography is critical to the proper diagnosis of ectopic pregnancies. If the patient has a serum β-hCG >6,000 mIU/mL, you should be able to visualize an intrauterine pregnancy using abdominal ultrasound scanning. Pregnancies can be identified much earlier using transvaginal ultrasound (Fig. 13-2). The discriminatory zone is the range of serum β-hCG values at which you can identify a uterine pregnancy using transvaginal ultrasound with >95% sensitivity. At most institutions, the approved discriminatory zone for serum β-hCG ranges between 1,500 and 2,500 mIU/mL.

Treatment

If a patient is not hemodynamically stable, the treatment is to first stabilize the patient. This consists of obtaining IV access with two large-bore IV needles. Resuscitation with IV fluids should begin until packed red blood cells are available. A Foley catheter should be placed in the bladder to maintain accurate urine output. A type and crossmatch for the number of necessary units of packed red blood cells should be performed. Simultaneously, the patient should be taken emergently to the operating room for surgical management of the ectopic pregnancy.

EXTENDED IN-HOSPITAL MANAGEMENT

There are several treatment modalities for ectopic pregnancy. The treatment of choice depends on the stability of the patient (Fig. 13-3). Management can be divided into surgical and medical.

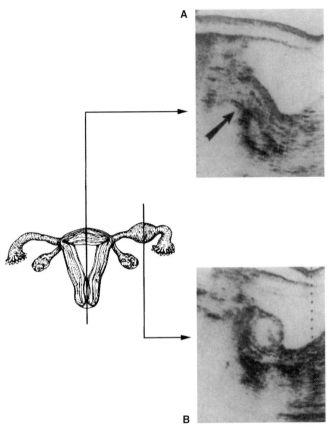

FIGURE 13-2: Transvaginal ultrasound of an adnexal ectopic pregnancy.

Surgical Management

As you take the patient to the operating room for surgical intervention of an ectopic pregnancy, the two questions you should ask yourself are (a) What will be my surgical approach? and (b) Which technique will I use?

Surgical Approach

Surgery can be performed either by laparoscopy or laparotomy. The decision to proceed with one over the other should be made based on the stability of the patient as well as the physician's technical ability to perform both procedures.

Laparoscopy

In a hemodynamically stable patient, laparoscopy is preferred to laparotomy. It is a minimally invasive approach that allows fast recovery for the patient.

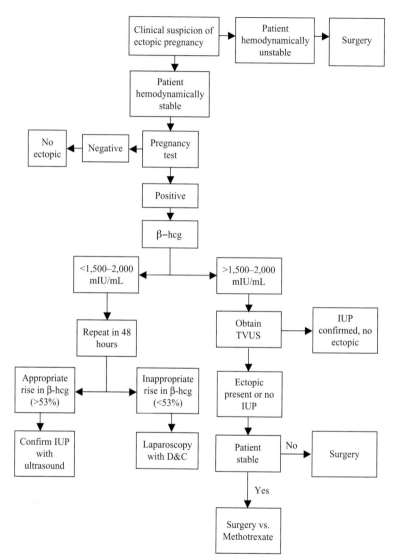

FIGURE 13-3: Algorithm for the diagnosis and treatment of ectopic pregnancy. IUP, intrauterine pregnancy; TVUS, transvaginal ultrasound.

However, the disadvantage of this approach is difficulty in controlling bleeding, which creates issues with visualization.

Laparotomy

Laparotomy is the recommended approach for a hemodynamically unstable patient. It allows for maximum exposure and great visualization, which allows quick access to the ectopic pregnancy in order to control bleeding.

Surgical Technique

Once the surgical approach has been decided, the surgical technique must be determined. The various techniques include salpingostomy or salpingectomy. The surgical technique is decided upon based on the location of the ectopic pregnancy as well as the size of the ectopic pregnancy.

Salpingostomy

This procedure involves making a linear incision in the antimesenteric border of the fallopian tube over the area where the ectopic pregnancy is suspected (Fig. 13-4). The products are then removed from the tube. The ostomy is left open to heal by secondary intention. This option is reserved for those patients with an abnormal contralateral fallopian tube.

Salpingectomy

This procedure involves removal of the entire fallopian tube or the portion of the tube that contains the ectopic pregnancy. This option is reserved for those patients with a large or ruptured ectopic pregnancy in whom the tube cannot be saved.

Medical Management

Medical management is becoming an increasingly viable option for the treatment of a stable ectopic pregnancy. This is because of the ability to diagnose ectopic pregnancies early in their development. One primary advantage to medical therapy is the ability to treat ectopic pregnancies in an outpatient setting. Medical management is achieved using the drug methotrexate, which inhibits dihydrofolate reductase and therefore DNA synthesis. Because methotrexate targets rapidly dividing cells, side effects are mostly related to the gastrointestinal tract and the bone marrow. Side effects are dose-related. Some of the severe side effects are ulcerative stomatitis, severe diarrhea, thrombocytopenia, and severe anemia. The more common side effects are nausea, vomiting, abdominal discomfort, diarrhea, and hair loss.

There are several relative and absolute contraindications to methotrexate treatment of ectopic pregnancy (6):

- Absolute contraindications
  - Breast-feeding
  - Evidence of immunodeficiency

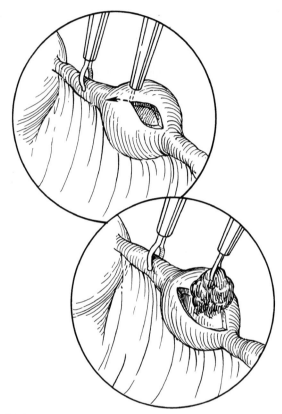

FIGURE 13-4: An incision is made into the antimesenteric border of the fallopian tube over the site of the suspected ectopic pregnancy. The products are removed. The salpingostomy site is allowed to heal by secondary intention.

- Alcoholism or liver disease
- Preexisting blood dyscrasias
- Sensitivity to methotrexate
- Active pulmonary disease
- Peptic ulcer disease
- Hepatic, renal, or hematologic dysfunction
- Relative contraindications
  - Gestational sac ≥3.5 cm
  - Embryonic cardiac motion

Methotrexate can be given through one of two regimens: single-dose or multidose therapy. Success rates with methotrexate have been reported between 67% and 92% (7).

DISPOSITION

Discharge Goals

After surgical intervention, patients are discharged using standard postoperative markers. Hemodynamic stability and the return of gastrointestinal function are the two goals that must be achieved before a patient can safely be discharged from the hospital. Medically treated patients must be counseled on the possible side effects of methotrexate. In addition, they should be informed to expect an initial increase in abdominal pain. This is thought to be due to extrusion of blood from the tube during the disintegration of the pregnancy and/or tubal distention. However, patients must also be aware that if they have a further increase in abdominal pain, they should seek immediate medical attention because this could be a sign of treatment failure.

Outpatient Care

After providing management for an ectopic pregnancy, it is important to follow weekly β-hCG levels to prepregnancy levels. Patients are encouraged to use a reliable contraceptive method while the hormone level is being followed. If the β-hCG level begins to rise, a chronic ectopic pregnancy should be suspected and may require repeat treatment. Also, patients with an Rh-negative blood type should be administered RhoGAM postoperatively to prevent isoimmunization in future pregnancies.

WHAT YOU NEED TO REMEMBER

- An ectopic pregnancy is a pregnancy that implants in a location other than the endometrium.
- Patients with a history of pelvic infection, tubal surgery, and ectopic pregnancy are at increased risk for the development of ectopic pregnancy.
- The triad of symptoms for a patient with an ectopic pregnancy is abdominal pain, amenorrhea, and irregular vaginal bleeding.
- Diagnosis can be made by combining clinical suspicion with an elevated β-hCG level and no evidence of intrauterine pregnancy on ultrasound.
- Treatment can be either medical or surgical, depending on the hemodynamic status of the patient and the size of the ectopic pregnancy.
- Surgical management can be performed via laparoscopy or laparotomy.
- Medical management is with methotrexate.

REFERENCES

1. Gabbe S, Niebyl JR, Simpson JL. *Obstetrics: Normal and Problem Pregnancies.* 4th ed. New York, NY: Churchill Livingstone; 2002.
2. Menon S, Sammel MD, Vichnin M, et al. Risk factors for ectopic pregnancy: a comparison between adults and adolescent women. *J Pediatr Adolesc Gynecol.* 2007;20:181–185.
3. Centers for Disease Control and Prevention. Current Trends Ectopic Pregnancy: United States, 1990-1992. *MMWR Morb Mortal Weekly Rep.* 1995;44(3):46–48.
4. Lobo R. Ectopic pregnancy—etiology, pathology, diagnosis, management, fertility, prognosis. In: Stevencher MA, Droegemueller W, Herbst A, et al, eds. *Comprehensive Gynecology.* 5th ed. St. Louis, MO: Mosby; 2001:389–419.
5. Mukul L, Teal SB. Current management of ectopic pregnancy. *Obstet Gynecol Clin North Am.* 2007;34:403–419.
6. American College of Obstetricians and Gynecologists. ACOG practice bulletin number 3, December 1998: clinical management and guidelines for obstetrician-gynecologists. *Int J Gynaecol Obstet.* 1999;65(1):97–103.
7. Barnhart KT, Gosman G, Ashby R, et al. The medical management of ectopic pregnancy: a meta-analysis comparing "single dose" and "multidose" regimens. *Obstet Gynecol.* 2003;101:778–784.

SUGGESTED READINGS

Kumar V, Fausto N, Abbas A. *Robbins and Cotran Pathologic Basis of Disease.* 7th ed. St Louis, MO: Saunders; 2004.
Murray H, Baakdah H, Bardell T, et al. Diagnosis and treatment of ectopic pregnancy. *CMAJ.* 2005;173(8):905–912.
Schorge J, Schaffer J, Halvorson L, et al. Ectopic pregnancy. In: *Williams Gynecology.* New York: McGraw-Hill; 2008:157–174.

Abortion

👪 **THE PATIENT ENCOUNTER**

The next patient waiting to see you is a 24-year-old woman (G5P4) who had a positive pregnancy test at home and now has been having vaginal bleeding with abdominal cramping for 2 days. The first day of her last menstrual period was 5 weeks ago. The patient reports seeing some small clots but denies passing anything resembling tissue. She is feeling a bit dizzy, but does not indicate any other symptoms.

OVERVIEW

Definitions

Spontaneous abortion, also referred to as a *miscarriage*, is defined by the World Health Organization (WHO) as a loss of pregnancy before viability (~20 weeks), with the fetus weighing <500 g.

There are many subtypes of abortion, which can be diagnosed by physical exam and sonographic evaluation (1) (Table 14-1):

- *Threatened abortion* is defined as vaginal bleeding with evidence of an intrauterine pregnancy on sonogram or Doppler exam, and a closed cervix on physical exam.
- *Missed abortion*, also referred to as *blighted ovum*, *anembryonic pregnancy*, or *embryonic* or *fetal death*, is defined as a nonviable pregnancy, confirmed by sonogram, without passage of fetal tissue for a prolonged period of time, and a closed cervix on physical exam. The uterus may also measure smaller than expected on the bimanual exam.
- *Completed abortion* is defined as passage of all fetal and placental tissue, usually expelled together early in gestation without complications, and a closed cervix with minimal bleeding on exam.
- *Inevitable abortion* is defined by a dilated or open cervical os without the passage of fetal tissue with variable amounts of bleeding on exam.
- *Incomplete abortion* is defined as the partial passing of fetal tissue, active bleeding, and an open cervical os (Fig. 14-1).
- *Septic abortion* is defined as having an incomplete abortion or recent surgical procedure (vacuum aspiration, dilation and curettage, dilation and evacuation) with signs of systemic infection, including fever, tachycardia, hypotension, tachypnea, and uterine tenderness.

TABLE 14-1
Types of Spontaneous Abortion

Category	Cervix	Bleeding on Examination	Pregnancy on Sonogram
Threatened	Closed	Variable	Yes
Missed	Closed	Variable	Yes
Complete	Closed	Minimal	No
Inevitable	Open	Variable	Yes
Incomplete	Open	Actively bleeding	Variable
Septic	Closed/open	Yes	Variable

Recurrent abortion is defined as three or more consecutive spontaneous abortions.

Pathophysiology
Most spontaneous abortions are due to chromosomal or genetic abnormalities (1). Another process associated with pregnancy loss is inherited thrombophilias. The exact pathophysiology is not known but is suspected to be due to microemboli that alter the gestation's ability to develop.

Epidemiology
According to WHO, data from developed countries suggest that about 15% of all clinically recognized pregnancies result in abortion (2). Also, >80% of abortions occur in the first 12 weeks of pregnancy (1). Commonly occurring vaginal spotting or heavier bleeding during early gestation may persist for days or weeks, and may affect one of four or five pregnant women. Overall, approximately half of these pregnancies will abort, although the risk is substantially lower if fetal cardiac activity can be obtained (1). When cardiac activity has been demonstrated, the miscarriage rate is reduced to 2% to 3% in asymptomatic low-risk women (3).

CLINICAL PEARL
Nearly 15% of all recognized pregnancies result in an abortion. Women with first-trimester bleeding are at high risk for miscarriage until cardiac activity is obtained.

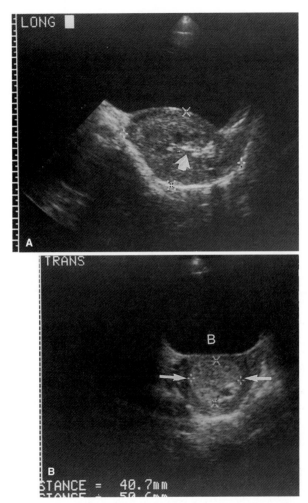

FIGURE 14-1: **Appearance of the Uterus after Incomplete Abortion. A:** Longitudinal scan shows retained placental products (*arrow*). **B:** Transverse scan shows the retained products of conception (*arrows*). Notice the position of the bladder (B) above the uterus.

Etiology

The most common cause of spontaneous abortion, accounting for approximately 50% of cases, is fetal chromosomal abnormalities. Autosomal trisomies (trisomy 21, 16, 18, 13) and monosomy (45, X) are the most and second most frequently identified chromosomal anomalies, respectively (1). In about two thirds of early pregnancy failures, there is anatomic evidence of defective placentation (3). Possible risk factors for spontaneous abortion include the following: previous spontaneous abortion, advanced maternal age, low folic acid intake, smoking, high alcohol consumption, cocaine use, nonsteroidal anti-inflammatory drug use, caffeine use, low maternal weight, and obesity. There are also many medical conditions that predispose a woman to having a spontaneous abortion, such as uncontrolled diabetes, thyroid disorders, and thrombophilias.

ACUTE MANAGEMENT AND WORKUP

The acute management of abortions is as much counseling as it is surgical intervention. The hardest aspect of the acute management of abortions is reassuring the patient that the event is not related to anything she did.

The First 15 Minutes

A trained physician should be able to quickly evaluate, diagnose, counsel, and provide prompt medical or surgical care for a pregnant woman who is in her first trimester and has vaginal bleeding. With some conditions that are emergent, it is important to have a routine for evaluating these patients to avoid preventable life-threatening complications.

Initial Assessment

Determining your patient's condition indicates the level of care you need to immediately provide for your patient. Your assessment should be focused to obtain the following needed information:

1. What is the first day of her last menstrual period and has she seen a doctor for prenatal care? If so, did she have a sonogram to confirm her pregnancy or has she previously heard the fetal heartbeat?
2. How is the patient feeling? Is she experiencing fevers, chills, abdominal pain, dizziness, shortness of breath, or palpitations?
3. When did her bleeding begin? How long has she been bleeding? How many thin or thick sanitary pads is she using per hour and per day?
4. Has she passed anything resembling tissue at home? If so, it is recommended to have the patient bring any tissue for pathologic evaluation.

Admission Criteria and Level of Care Criteria

Rapid assessment of your patient's overall condition, including vital signs and the amount of blood loss, is crucial in the first minutes of the patient's presentation. You must then determine whether or not the patient is stable.

Unstable Patients

Unstable patients are those with an altered mental status, fevers, hypotension, tachycardia, tachypnea, and noticeable bleeding. For these patients, perform the following tasks:

1. Start a large-bore intravenous (IV) lines for fluid or blood resuscitation. If the patient is tachycardic or hypotensive, begin giving a bolus of IV lactated Ringer or normal saline. Patients with signs of significant blood loss should be typed and crossmatched immediately for blood products.
2. Patients who are febrile should have blood cultures drawn from two different sites and given Tylenol (1 g) by mouth.
3. Obtain a focused history and perform a physical exam.
4. Perform a sterile speculum exam and determine how much bleeding is present, whether tissue is present, and if the cervix is open or closed.
5. If the cervix is open and tissue is in the cervical os or vagina, removing it with ringed forceps may alleviate the bleeding. If the patient continues to bleed heavily, she probably has retained products of conception and needs treatment for an incomplete abortion.
6. All material in the vault must be examined for the presence of products of conception. Send all tissue for pathologic evaluation.
7. Perform a bimanual exam to determine how far along the pregnancy is, and evaluate if the uterine fundus is tender and if the patient feels febrile internally.
8. If possible, obtain a transvaginal or abdominal sonogram to assist with making a diagnosis.

Stable Patients

For a patient who has no evidence of active bleeding, perform the following tasks:

1. First, obtain a urine pregnancy test to confirm that the patient indeed has a pregnancy, and draw the necessary blood tests.
2. Obtain a detailed history and perform a physical exam, including a speculum exam.
3. If your patient has a closed cervix during the speculum exam, include a gonococcal and chlamydial culture or DNA probe, and a microscopic wet mount exam to rule out any active infection.
4. Listen for fetal heartbeat and obtain a transvaginal or abdominal sonogram to aide the diagnosis.

The First Few Hours

After determining your patient's condition and diagnosis, the next step is to develop a management plan.

History

A large part of the history related to developing a management plan relates to the patient's preference and expectations. Assuming the patient is hemodynamically stable, a highly desired pregnancy may warrant observation with re-evaluation in 48 hours even if termination is inevitable.

Physical Examination

The most important aspect of the physical is the speculum exam. Assessment of cervical dilatation offers insight into the need for immediate surgical intervention. Any products of conception should be sent for pathologic evaluation for confirmation.

Labs and Tests to Consider

The main lab tests that you should order are similar to those collected when a patient initiates prenatal care. These tests include:

- Blood type (A, B, O)
- Rh status
- Antibody status
- Type and crossmatch
- Complete blood count with differential
- Human immunodeficiency virus, rapid plasma reagin, and hepatitis B surface antigen
- Quantitative beta subunit of human chorionic gonadotropin (β-hCG)

All Rh-negative women with a negative antibody screen must be treated with anti-D-immunoglobulin within 72 hours of the vaginal bleeding, abdominal trauma, or spontaneous abortion, regardless of management, to prevent isoimmunization.

Imaging

Sonography is the single best tool for the diagnosis and evaluation of early pregnancy with vaginal bleeding. Serial β-hCG tests may be used in combination with sonography for the evaluation of fetal viability. With a β-hCG level of 1,500 to 2,000 IU/mL (quantity varies by institution), an intrauterine gestation should be seen using transvaginal ultrasound. If no intrauterine pregnancy is observed, one must rule out the presence of an ectopic pregnancy.

Most pregnancies that lead to an abortion will have transvaginal sonographic evidence of an anembryonic pregnancy, revealed by a gestational sac measuring at least 17 to 20 mm without a fetal pole or yolk sac. When a fetal pole is present and measures more than 5 to 10 mm, the absence of cardiac activity is reliably diagnostic for embryonic death (4). Other sonographic signs of impending abortion are an irregularly shaped gestational sac, a slow fetal heartbeat, and irregular blood flow in the gestational sac (Fig. 14-2). If

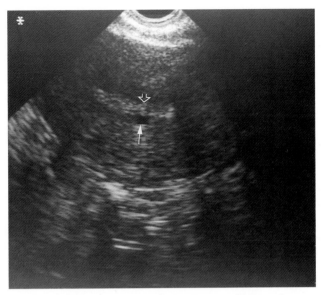

FIGURE 14-2: **Normal 3- to 4-week Gestation.** Ultrasound examination shows the small gestational sac (*solid arrow*) attached to the thickened uterine wall (*open arrow*).

you are unsure of the diagnosis of a missed abortion, it is always safe to have the patient return in 2 to 7 days for additional imaging and laboratory evaluation. It is also important to recognize the difference between a true gestational sac and the pseudogestational sac, which can be found on sonography when an ectopic pregnancy is present.

Treatment

The differential diagnosis for a first-trimester pregnancy with bleeding, in order of concern, is as follows: ectopic pregnancy; hydatidiform mole, incomplete abortion, impending abortion; pathology related to the cervix, vagina, or uterus (polyps, fibroids); and physiologic bleeding (implantation). Again, you should always first rule out the possibility of an ectopic pregnancy.

Formal treatment of abortions depends on the diagnosis and the stability of the clinical situation (Table 14-2).

Incomplete abortions and septic abortions are usually managed in a hospital setting with surgical treatment, although more studies have been published recently highlighting in-office procedures and the medical management of incomplete abortions. All septic patients should be surgically managed, treated with IV antibiotics, and given supportive care, including IV fluids and antipyretics.

TABLE 14-2
Management of Spontaneous Abortion

Category	Management
Threatened	Pelvic rest, repeat sonogram
Incomplete	Misoprostol, manual vacuum aspiration, suction curettage, sharp curettage (with or without dilation)
Inevitable	Expectant, misoprostol, vacuum aspiration or suction curettage or sharp curettage
Complete	Pelvic rest, family planning
Missed	Expectant, misoprostol, dilation with vacuum aspiration or suction curettage or sharp curettage
Septic	Immediate surgical management (vacuum aspiration or suction curettage or sharp curettage), intravenous broad-spectrum antibiotics, supportive care

Surgical treatments include: (a) manual vacuum aspiration using a reusable 60-mL syringe attached to a cannula, which provides continuous suction force; (b) electric vacuum aspiration, which provides continuous suction force; and (c) sharp curettage. The benefits of surgical management include convenient timing for the patient and high success rates, ranging from 93% to 100%, with most studies reporting success rates at or above 98%. Surgical risks, although relatively rare, include infection, uterine perforation, cervical trauma, and uterine adhesions (5). Anesthetic risks will vary depending on the type of anesthesia used and the duration of the procedure.

> **CLINICAL PEARL**
>
> *When performing a surgical abortion, patients should receive doxycycline, 100 mg orally 1 hour prior to the procedure and 200 mg after the procedure, for antibiotic prophylaxis. If your patient is allergic to doxycycline, it is recommended to use metronidazole 500 mg orally twice a day for 5 days.*

EXTENDED IN-HOSPITAL MANAGEMENT

Abortions are typically managed in outpatient settings. The only patients who require extended in-hospital management are those who develop a septic abortion or who are symptomatic from acute blood loss anemia. Broad-spectrum IV antibiotics and appropriate blood products, respectively, are used to treat these patients.

DISPOSITION
Discharge Goals
Broad-spectrum IV antibiotic treatment is continued until the patient has been afebrile for 48 hours with a downward trending white blood count. Upon discharge, many institutions regularly prescribe a 10-day course of oral broad-spectrum antibiotics such as doxycycline to further treat infection. Patients should be instructed to abstain from intercourse to prevent infection. Patients should be prescribed oral iron sulfate to help replenish their blood stores secondary to the acute blood loss.

Outpatient Care
For a majority of your patients, you will be able to manage the abnormal pregnancy in an outpatient setting. The treatment options primarily depend on your patient's preference.

Medical Management
Medical management of missed, inevitable, or incomplete abortions includes insertion of four misoprostol 200-mcg tablets into the posterior fornix of the vagina to aid with uterine contractions and expulsion of the uterine contents. Close follow-up with serial sonograms is needed to document a completed abortion; repeating the misoprostol in 72 hours may be necessary in some patients (3). Hygroscopic dilators, such as laminarias and Lamicel, can be inserted into the cervix overnight to allow the cervix to soften and dilate without the brute force and risk of cervical trauma related to manual dilation. The patient can return to the office or hospital on the following day for a surgical procedure.

Expectant Management
Patients diagnosed with a threatened or missed abortion should be advised appropriately and can be safely discharged with close follow-up care and strong advisement to return to the emergency setting if they experience severe bleeding (soaking more than two regular pads per hour for 2 hours), the passing of any tissue, severe abdominal pain, fever, or any other emergent condition. The patient should be instructed to take prenatal vitamins and abstain from intercourse or inserting anything into her vagina. Bed rest has never been scientifically proven to help prevent abortion, and patients should be instructed to perform at an activity level with which they are comfortable (1).

According to a review by Nanda et al. (5), patients expectantly managed have an increased amount of pain and bleeding, as well as an increase in the number of days of bleeding (approximately 2 more days). These patients also have a significantly lower rate of pelvic infection. However, approximately 10% of these patients will need surgical intervention and an additional 11% will choose to have a surgical procedure to eliminate the bleeding and waiting time.

Family Planning

Ovulation may resume as soon as 2 weeks after resolution of the abortion (1). Patients should be encouraged to refrain from intercourse for 4 weeks to prevent infection, should continue taking prenatal vitamins daily if they desire pregnancy, and should be given proper birth control to prevent an unwanted pregnancy.

WHAT YOU NEED TO REMEMBER

- The proper evaluation and management of first-trimester vaginal bleeding is important in terms of both emergent medical care and influences on the ongoing and future needs of the mother and baby.
- The rapid clinical assessment of patients with a positive pregnancy test and vaginal bleeding is necessary to determine the need for medical or surgical management.
- Be sure to rule out the possibility of an ectopic pregnancy.
- This visit may be the patient's first receipt of obstetric care. As the physician, your role may include counseling a woman about the importance of early prenatal care, improving the outcome of mother and child, and providing services to save the life of your patient.

REFERENCES

1. Cunningham G, Leveno K, Bloom S, et al. *Williams Obstetrics*. 22nd ed. New York, NY: McGraw-Hill; 2005:232–239.
2. Weeks A. Expectant care versus surgical treatment for miscarriage: RHL commentary (last revised: 15 December 2006). *The WHO Reproductive Health Library*. Geneva: World Health Organization.
3. Robledo C, Zhang J, Troendle J, et al. Clinical indicators for success of misoprostol treatment after early pregnancy failure. *Int J Gynecol Obstet*. 2007;99:46–51.
4. Gabbe SG, Niebyl JR, Simpson JL. *Obstetrics: Normal and Problem Pregnancies*, 5th ed. New York, NY: Churchill Livingstone; 2007.
5. Nanda K, Peloggi A, Grimes D, et al. Expectant care versus surgical treatment for miscarriage. *Cochrane Database Syst Rev*. 2006;(2):CD003518.

Vaginal Infections

THE PATIENT ENCOUNTER

A 32-year-old divorced woman (G2P2) presents with a 4-day history of vaginal discharge. She has been in a new relationship for the past 6 months and has recently become sexually active again. She is concerned because the discharge smells "fishy," particularly at times of sexual activity. She is embarrassed and afraid that her new partner will notice, so she has begun to avoid intimacy. She has an otherwise unremarkable medical history.

OVERVIEW

Definition

Vulvovaginitis, or infection of the vagina and vulva with inflammation, is defined as the spectrum of conditions that cause vulvovaginal symptoms such as itching, burning, irritation, and abnormal discharge. Vaginosis refers to vulvovaginal symptoms caused by the overgrowth of vaginal flora *without* a corresponding inflammatory response.

Pathophysiology

The vaginal microbial milieu is complex and depends on many endogenous and exogenous factors. A pH of 3.5 to 4.5 is important in suppressing the growth of pathogenic organisms. Estrogen is the most important endogenous factor and exerts both a lowering effect on pH and an inhibitory effect on anaerobic bacteria. In estrogen-deficient states, such as the prepubertal and postmenopausal periods, the pH of the vagina usually is elevated. In the reproductive years, lactobacilli, the dominant vaginal flora, flourish under the influence of estrogen and contribute to the maintenance of a low pH by producing lactic acid. Exogenous factors that may alter the vaginal ecosystem include menstruation, parturition, genital tract surgery, antibiotic therapy, foreign bodies, douching, and the presence of semen.

Epidemiology

Vulvovaginitis is one of most common problems encountered by gynecologists and affects all age groups, from young girls to elderly women. Unfortunately, frequent self-diagnosis and treatment with over-the-counter preparations causes some difficulty in monitoring epidemiologic trends.

Etiology

The most common causes of symptomatic vaginal infection are bacterial vaginosis (BV), vulvovaginal candidiasis, and trichomoniasis. Vaginitis is also associated with sexually transmitted diseases. Excluding human papillomavirus, genital herpes from herpes simplex virus 1 (HSV1) or 2 (HSV2) has become the most common sexually transmitted infection among women. Undiagnosed vaginitis occurs in up to 72% of women, with symptoms caused by a broad array of conditions including atrophic vaginitis, vulvar dermatosis, and vulvodynia.

ACUTE MANAGEMENT AND WORKUP

Symptomatic vaginal infection is typically a mild condition that is almost exclusively managed in a primary care or office setting. As a result, an acute or emergent phase is often not present. However, severe pain, severe dysuria, urinary retention, or serious complications of herpes may cause patients to visit the emergency room.

The First 15 Minutes

A focused clinical visit for this complaint should take about 15 minutes in its entirety. If the patient appears uncomfortable or ill, a brief initial assessment for complications may be necessary.

Initial Assessment

The initial assessment should focus on the following four aspects:

1. Patient History
   - Acute suprapubic pain with inability to urinate suggests acute retention.
   - Constitutional symptoms such as fevers, malaise, myalgias, and headache may signal primary herpes or more severe disease
2. Observation of the Patient
   - Disorientation, mental status changes, or focal neurologic symptoms or signs suggest herpes with CNS involvement.
3. Vital Signs
   - An elevated temperature and heart rate may suggest a systemic infection.
4. Pelvic Exam
   - Vulvar vesicles suggest herpes. Lesions with surrounding erythema and induration suggest a superimposed bacterial infection.

Admission Criteria and Level of Care Criteria

Patients with severe HSV disease or complications, such as disseminated infection or CNS involvement, should be hospitalized with supportive care and intravenous antiviral therapy. Urethral catheter placement with outpatient management is appropriate for patients in urinary retention or with severe dysuria. All other patients can be safely managed in an outpatient setting.

The First Few Hours

The overwhelming majority of patients with vulvovaginitis are managed in an outpatient clinic setting. In most cases, clinical presentation and investigative findings are unique for each infection. The salient features of history, exam, and diagnosis for the common causes of vaginal infection can be found in Table 15-1.

> **CLINICAL PEARL**
>
> *To make the diagnosis of bacterial vaginosis, you must meet Amsel's criteria. Diagnosis requires three of the following four symptoms or signs: (i) homogeneous, thin, white discharge that smoothly coats the vaginal walls; (ii) presence of clue cells on microscopic examination; (iii) pH of vaginal fluid >4.5; and (iv) a fishy odor of vaginal discharge before or after addition of 10% potassium hydroxide (i.e., the whiff test).*

History

A full history should be obtained that focuses on the spectrum of vaginal symptoms, including discharge, odor, itching, irritation, burning, swelling, dyspareunia, and dysuria. Questions about symptom location, duration, menstrual variations, precipitating factors, and response to prior treatment can yield important insight into the potential cause. A personal sexual history, partner symptomatology, and accompanying psychological and psychosexual dysfunction are also important, especially if symptoms are chronic or recurrent. When itching and burning are prominent symptoms, the patient should be questioned about the use of irritating substances such as soaps, bath additives, douches, and laundry detergents.

Candidiasis

Pregnancy, diabetes, immunosuppression, and antibiotic use are risk factors for a candidal infection. With recurrent disease, underlying conditions should be considered, particularly poorly controlled diabetes or human immunodeficiency virus (HIV).

Bacterial Vaginosis

Bacterial vaginosis is a polymicrobial infection marked by the overgrowth of anaerobic organisms. Bacterial vaginosis has been associated with postabortal infection, postprocedural gynecologic infections, pelvic

TABLE 15-1

History, Physical Examination, and Diagnostic Findings of Common Vaginal Infections

Finding	Candidiasis	Bacterial Vaginosis	Trichomonas	Genital Herpes Simplex	Atrophic Vaginitis
History Pruritus	Yes	No	Yes	No	Yes
Discharge	Thick, white, curdy "cottage cheese"	Thin, grey/white	Thin, yellow-green to grey "frothy"	Profuse if cervix involved (atypical)	Thin, gray or serosanguineous
Odor	No	Offensive "fishy"	Offensive "rancid"	No	No
Erythema	Yes	No	Yes	No	No
Urinary symptoms	Dysuria	No	Dysuria	Dysuria	Urgency/frequency/UTI/incontinence
Dyspareunia	Yes	No	Yes	Yes	Yes
Other	Intense burning or soreness	Symptoms worse after intercourse or menses	Postcoital bleeding Intense burning	Pain/vesicles ulcers/fissures	May have other menopausal symptoms

Physical exam	Vulva/vagina inflamed, excoriations, **thick adherent plaquelike discharge.** May have satellite vulvar lesions	Watery discharge, **absence of inflammation**	Vulva/vagina inflamed. Punctuate cervical intra-epithelial hemorrhages. **"Strawberry cervix"**	Multiple small vulvar vesicles/ulcers. May have cervical lesions. Inguinal lymphadenopathy.	Vulva/vagina pale, thin, dry, smooth, shiny. May have vaginal erythema, contact bleeding, or laceration. Loss of rugae.
Diagnosis pH	<4.5	>4.5	>4.5	<4.5	>4.5
Microscopy	**KOH prep with yeast or pseudohyphae**	**Clue cells No leukocytes**	**Motile, flagellated organisms** and leukocytes	—	Parabasal, intermediate cells, loss of superficial cells, leukocytes
Other	—	**Positive amine "whiff" test**	—	Culture, serology, PCR	—
Criterion standard	Microscopy	Amsel's criteria	Microscopy	Viral culture	Microscopy

UTI, urinary tract infection; KOH, potassium hydroxide; PCR, polymerase chain reaction.

inflammatory disease (PID), infertility, and the acquisition of HIV and HSV2 infections.

Trichomoniasis

Trichomoniasis is caused by flagellated, motile, anaerobic protozoan that colonizes the urethra as well as the vagina. Infection is predominantly sexually transmitted, but may occur via fomites and has been shown to survive in hot tubs and swimming pools. Trichomoniasis has been associated with PID, endometritis, infertility, ectopic pregnancy, preterm birth, and is associated with facilitating HIV transmission.

Genital Herpes

Genital herpes is caused by HSV1 or HSV2 acquired by skin-to-skin contact or mucous membrane contact during periods of active virus shedding. First-episode infections are the most severe, with a flulike syndrome and frequent neurologic involvement. Given the variability of presentation, it is not possible to state on clinical grounds alone whether a particular episode is primary or recurrent, or which type is responsible.

Physical Examination

The physical exam begins with a thorough evaluation of the vulva for lesions, erythema, induration, and atrophy. Gentle separation of the labia will allow visualization of the urethra and introitus. The cervix and vaginal mucosa should be examined with a speculum for discharge, lesions, inflammation, and degree of estrogen effect. Samples should be obtained for vaginal pH, amine ("whiff") test, saline (wet mount), and 10% KOH microscopy. Relevant physical exam findings can be found in Table 15-1.

Labs and Tests to Consider

Microscopy is considered the standard test for vaginitis in clinical practice (Fig. 15-1). However, in certain circumstances, ancillary testing is indicated.

Cultures. Culture of vaginal secretions is the most sensitive and specific commercially available method to diagnose trichomoniasis and should be obtained in women in whom the diagnosis is suspected but not confirmed microscopically.

CLINICAL PEARL

Vaginal yeast cultures should be obtained for recurrent candidiasis or in women with multiple symptoms and a negative findings on microscopic wet mount.

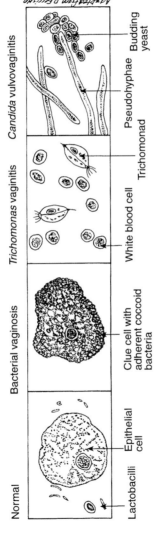

Normal

Bacterial vaginosis

Trichomonas vaginitis

Candida vulvovaginitis

Lactobacilli

Epithelial cell

Clue cell with adherent coccoid bacteria

White blood cell

Trichomonad

Pseudohyphae

Budding yeast

Adapted from D.Ferriso

FIGURE 15-1: Wet mount findings of vaginal secretions in women with vaginitis.

Gram Stain. In patients with symptoms suggestive of BV who do not fulfill Amsel's criteria, a Gram stain for Gram-negative rods characteristic of BV is considered the criterion standard for diagnosis.

DNA and Blood Tests. DNA tests or cultures for gonorrhea and chlamydia should be obtained in sexually active adolescents, other women at high risk, and patients with a purulent discharge, friable cervix, symptoms suggestive of PID, or leukocytes on microscopy. Patients with sexually transmitted diseases, recurrent symptoms, or in high-risk groups should be offered a full screen for other sexually transmitted infections, including HIV.

Biopsy. Vulvar skin or vulvar-vaginal epithelium biopsy may be indicated for unusual lesions, suspicion of a noninfective cause, or lesions or ulcers that do not respond to initial therapy.

Key Diagnostic Labs and Tests

With the exception of HSV, the cause of vaginal symptoms can usually be determined by pH and a wet mount microscopic evaluation of the discharge. However, recent intercourse, menses, sampling of cervical mucus, or recent treatment with medications can alter the pH of the vagina and affect the results. Table 15-1 includes the appropriate diagnostic tests.

Imaging

No imaging is necessary as the diagnosis is made on the basis of the history, physical exam, and microscopic and laboratory findings.

Treatment

General conservative measures for symptom relief include oral analgesia, topical anesthetic, saline baths, the avoidance of irritants, and abstinence. Typical treatment regimens and alternatives are shown in Table 15-2.

Candidiasis

In uncomplicated cases, topical or oral imidazoles are first-line therapy. Complicated cases are characterized by recurrence, severe disease, candidiasis not related to *Candida albicans*, or concurrent conditions such as uncontrolled diabetes, immunosuppression, and pregnancy. Most complicated cases respond to 7 to 14 days of azole therapy, with boric acid (600 mg vaginal suppositories every night × 14 days) reserved for treatment failures. The treatment of sex partners is not recommended, but can be considered in women with recurrent infections.

Bacterial Vaginosis

Treatment for BV before abortion or hysterectomy significantly decreases the risk of postoperative infectious complications, and helps to resolve

TABLE 15-2

Standard Treatment Regimens and Alternatives for Vaginal Infections

Disease	Standard Treatment	Alternative
Candidiasis Uncomplicated	• fluconazole 150 mg orally × 1 dose	• Azole intravaginal therapy 1–3 days
Complicated Severe	• Fluconazole 150 mg orally every 72 hours × 2 doses	• Azole intravaginal therapy 7–14 days
Recurrent	• Fluconazole 150 mg orally every 3 days × 3 doses	• Azole intravaginal therapy 7–14 days
Bacterial vaginosis	• Metronidazole 500 mg orally twice a day for 7 days *OR* • Metronidazole 0.75% gel 5 g intravaginal once a day for 5 days	• Clindamycin 2% cream 5 g. intravaginal at bedtime for 7 days *OR* • Clindamycin 300 mg orally twice a day for 7 days
Trichomoniasis	• Metronidazole 2 g orally × 1 dose *OR* • Tinidazole 2 g orally × 1 dose	• Metronidazole 500 mg orally twice a day for 7 days

(continued)

TABLE 15-2
Standard Treatment Regimens and Alternatives for Vaginal Infections (Continued)

Disease	Standard Treatment	Alternative
Genital herpes First episode	• Acyclovir 400 mg orally 3 times a day for 7–10 days **OR** • Famciclovir 250 mg orally 3 times a day for 7–10 days **OR** • Valacyclovir 1 g orally twice a day for 7–10 days	• Acyclovir 200 mg orally 5 times a day for 7–10 days
Recurrent	• Acyclovir 800 mg 3 times a day for 2 days **OR** • Acyclovir 400 mg orally 3 times a day for 5 days **OR**	• Famciclovir 125 mg orally twice a day for 3–5 days **OR** • Valacyclovir 500 mg orally twice a day for 3 days
Suppressive	• Acyclovir 400 mg orally twice a day **OR** • Famciclovir 250 mg orally twice a day **OR** • Valacyclovir 500 mg to 1 g once a day	• Acyclovir 200 mg orally 2 to 5 times a day
Atrophic vaginitis	• Local/systemic estrogen	• Water-based moisturizer/lubricant

concurrent mucopurulent cervicitis. Oral or vaginal metronidazole is first-line therapy and patients must be advised to avoid alcohol, as a disulfiram-like reaction may occur with both oral and topical treatments. There is no benefit to investigating or treating the male partner.

Trichomoniasis

Oral therapy is necessary to eradicate the organism from the urethra as well as the vagina. Metronidazole and tinidazole are the only oral medications available in the United States for the treatment of trichomoniasis. Both are equally efficacious and alcohol should be avoided for 24 hours after metronidazole and 72 hours after tinidazole. The patient should be advised to avoid unprotected intercourse during treatment, and partners should be treated.

Genital Herpes

Antiviral chemotherapy is the mainstay of treatment for symptomatic patients. For first-episode HSV infections, oral antiviral therapy should be started to reduce symptoms, as treatment does not eradicate the virus or reduce the risk, frequency, or severity of recurrences. Recurrent episodes can be treated with abstinence and conservative symptom relief, episodic drug therapy, or suppressive therapy.

EXTENDED IN-HOSPITAL MANAGEMENT

In-hospital management typically applies only to severe herpes symptoms or complications. Patients should receive intravenous antiviral therapy until clinical improvement is observed and complications are adequately treated.

DISPOSITION

Discharge Goals

Prior to discharge, patients should be afebrile and hemodynamically stable. Pain should be well controlled with oral medications, and the patient should be tolerating oral intake. If she is unable to void spontaneously, a catheter may be left in place. Overall clinical improvement with good response to treatment should be observed prior to discharge.

Outpatient Care

Continued outpatient care of vaginal infections is essentially restricted to persistent symptoms and recurrences. For candidiasis, BV, and trichomoniasis, no follow-up is necessary if symptoms resolve. For herpes infections, in severe cases, it may be prudent to monitor lesion resolution or response to therapy. In patients with atrophic vaginitis, follow-up visits to reassess symptoms should be considered. Follow-up visits should also be considered for education counseling, results disclosure, or further investigation in individuals who do not respond to therapy.

WHAT YOU NEED TO REMEMBER

- Vulvovaginitis is one of most common problems encountered by gynecologists in primary care, and it affects all age groups.
- The vaginal microbial milieu is complex and depends on many endogenous and exogenous factors, and alterations often cause infection.
- The most common causes of symptomatic vaginal infection are bacterial vaginosis, vulvovaginal candidiasis, and trichomoniasis.
- In most cases of infectious vulvovaginitis, the clinical presentation and investigative findings are unique for each infection. With the exception of herpes, the diagnosis can often be made with the history, the exam, pH testing, and microscopy.
- Most patients can be managed in a single visit without follow-up.
- Be sure you educate and counsel your patients about safe sex practices.

SUGGESTED READINGS

American College of Obstetricians and Gynecologists. ACOG practice bulletin number 72: vaginitis. *Obstet Gynecol.* 2006;107:1195–1206.

American College of Obstetricians and Gynecologists. *Precis: an Update in Obstetrics and Gynecology.* 3rd ed. Washington, DC: American College of Obstetricians and Gynecologists; 2006.

Centers for Disease Control and Prevention. Sexually transmitted diseases guidelines, 2006. *MMWR.* 2006;55(No.RR-11):14–54.

Eckert LO, Lentz GM. Infections of the lower genital tract. In: Katz VL, Lentz GM, Lobo RA, et al., eds. *Comprehensive Gynecology.* 5th ed. Philadelphia: Mosby, 2007:569–607.

Impey L. *Obstetrics and Gynaecology.* 1st ed. Oxford: Blackwell Science; 1999.

Smith RP. *Netter's Obstetrics, Gynecology, and Women's Health.* Teterboro: MediMedia, Inc; 2002.

Vulvar Lesions

A 45-year-old woman presents to your office complaining of a new rash in her pelvic area. She tells you that the issue has been present for the last 2 years but she never sought treatment because it did not bother her until now. This rash is starting to itch more and has been causing her to experience a significant amount of pain with intercourse.

OVERVIEW

Definition

Lesions of the vulva are common and are classified based on their gross appearance and histopathologic changes. The range of diseases from benign to precancerous to cancerous is wide, and unfortunately the characteristics tend to overlap, making their differentiation difficult. The most common vulvar lesions you will encounter include lichen simplex chronicus, lichen sclerosus, inflammatory diseases, solid tumors of the vulva, and cystic tumors of the vulva.

Pathophysiology

The skin of the vulva is unique and more permeable than any of the surrounding tissues. Vulvar skin is particularly vulnerable to friction and irritants. The sensitivity of vulvar skin can induce a chronic itch-scratch cycle, making the healing process more difficult.

Epidemiology

The embarrassing nature of vulvar lesions makes estimating the incidence of disease challenging. Patients tend to underreport problems, and clinicians often misdiagnose these issues. One of the most well-studied vulvar lesions, lichen sclerosus, has been found to affect approximately 0.5% of all postmenopausal women, with a tendency toward white women.

Etiology

In general, vulvar lesions can originate from factors intrinsic or extrinsic to the vulvar skin environment. Hormonal and autoimmune theories have been suggested for predisposing women to lichen sclerosus. Extrinsic factors include inflammation due to an allergic irritant, bacterial or fungal infection, trauma, and even Bartholin's gland ductal obstruction, which leads to mucous retention.

ACUTE MANAGEMENT AND WORKUP

Pain and infection are the two most common reasons for an acute evaluation of a vulvar lesion. If the lesion is identified in a timely manner, outpatient therapy is appropriate and effective. The reality is that patient embarrassment leads to delayed presentation of these lesions and in-hospital management becomes necessary.

The First 15 Minutes

When you have a patient complaining of severe pelvic pain, the most important decision to make in the first 15 minutes is whether the patient has a surgical emergency. A vulvar lesion secondary to trauma may be an external manifestation of retroperitoneal bleeding. Necrotizing fasciitis of the vulva is another surgical emergency in which a delay in treatment could lead to significant morbidity and even mortality in your patient.

Initial Assessment

If you are consulted by a patient with an acute vulvar lesion, a quick review of your patient's vital signs, past medical history (especially diabetes), and the events preceding the visit will help you prioritize whether in-hospital or outpatient care is appropriate.

Admission Criteria and Level of Care Criteria

The three conditions that should heighten your level of care are (i) concern about impending sepsis, (ii) hemodynamic instability from bleeding, and (iii) pain uncontrolled by oral agents. An appropriate understanding of the underlying process will allow you to temper the manifesting symptoms and properly treat the disease process.

The First Few Hours

After you have made your initial assessment, the focus of the next few hours is getting a more detailed history, looking for risk factors that you can treat. Except for infectious vulvar lesions, the treatment course can take weeks and requires patience from both you and your patient. A careful history can help make the diagnosis correctly.

History

There are two key components to taking a history in relation to vulvar lesions: carefully characterizing the symptoms of the lesion and looking for a source of irritation. Characterization of vulvar lesions is similar to the classic history for pain—how long has the lesion been there, what makes it better, what makes it worse, has the patient ever had a similar lesion, what treatments has your patient tried, what are the other symptoms (burning, itching, drainage, fevers), and has the lesion changed in appearance? Local irritants can also lead to the chronic itch-scratch cycle, which exacerbates the symptoms. The source of these irritants can be anything from laundry detergent to topical medicines to the chemicals in hygiene products. Pay attention to any new products or habits. Finally, some systemic diseases (such as Crohn disease) can include vulvar manifestations.

Physical Examination

Each vulvar lesion has a particular characteristic that helps clinically define the disease (Table 16-1). A systematic assessment of the external genitalia with documentation of the findings allows you to track the progress of the lesion. In addition, it is important to perform a complete skin survey, including the buccal mucosa (as seen with lichen planus).

Another useful tool to use during your physical examination is to draw the lesion in relation to the patients normal anatomy in your patient's chart using a schematic similar to Figure 16-1. Depending on the sophistication of your medical records, a digital photograph of the lesion is an excellent way to document over time the progress of your treatment.

Labs and Tests to Consider

The diagnosis of vulvar lesions rarely relies on laboratory findings. The one test that is critical for the diagnosis of persistent vulvar lesions unresponsive to therapy is a Keyes punch biopsy (Fig. 16-2).

CLINICAL PEARL

Any vulvar area that possesses thickened epithelium, ulceration, necrosis, or persistent pain/puritis warrants a biopsy. In general, a 3- to 4-mm biopsy specimen is sufficient to make the correct diagnosis.

Treatment

As you are trying to clarify the diagnosis of your patient's vulvar lesion, you have the opportunity to teach your patient about good vulvar hygiene as outlined by the International Society for the Study of Vulvovaginal Disease (www.issvd.org). When washing the vulvar tissue, your patient should use plain warm water. Many of the soaps and shower gels are too harsh for the tissue and can cause more irritation. Do not use a hair dryer after washing;

TABLE 16-1

Summary of Common Vulvar Lesions

Category	Diagnosis	Defining Characteristics	First-Line Treatment Options
Nonneoplastic diseases	Lichen simplex chronicus	Excoriations, erythematous skin	Topical steroids, restore skin barrier
	Lichen sclerosus	Porcelain-white papules, forms a figure-8 or hourglass shape	Ultrapotent topical steroids
Inflammatory diseases	Contact dermatitis	Localized erythema with vesicles	Remove offending agent; avoid scratching
	Intertrigo	Fissuring in genitocrural folds	Drying agents (cornstarch) with mild steroids
	Lichen planus	Flat-topped, shiny polygon papules; oral involvement	Ultrapotent topical steroids, with or without oral retinoids
	Hidradenitis suppurativa	Recurrent papule lesions in intertriginous area; coalescence of nodules with abscess formation	Oral antibiotics; warm compresses

Solid tumors	Acrochordon	Skin tag	Removal if symptomatic
	fibroma	on labia majora; approximately 1-8 cm	Surgical removal
Cystic tumors	Bartholin's gland duct cyst	Unilateral; tender; lower vestibular area	I&D, marsupialization
	Skene's gland enlargement	Enlargement of gland at distal urethra	Excision

I&D, incision and drainage.

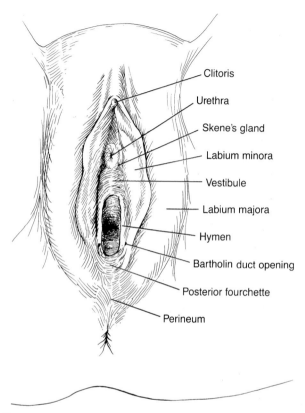

FIGURE 16-1: External female genitalia.

gently pad dry the outer skin. Cotton undergarments washed in a mild detergent are advisable, and at night your patient could consider wearing a skirt around the house with no underwear to avoid problems with friction. Finally, patients should never use products such as deodorants, douches, or other cosmetic/cleaning products in the vulvovaginal area.

Table 16-1 helps summarize the first-line treatments for the most common vulvar lesions you will encounter in your practice.

EXTENDED IN-HOSPITAL MANAGEMENT

Infectious and traumatic vulvar lesions are the main sources of pathology that require extended in-hospital therapy. Intravenous antibiotics can help

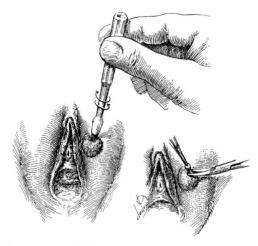

FIGURE 16-2: Keyes punch biopsy.

treat any superimposed bacterial and fungal infections. Local skin care is helpful in treating women with traumatic lesions. Both require daily observation for signs of improvement to confirm that the prescribed therapy is working.

DISPOSITION

Discharge Goals

If your patient has an infectious vulvar lesion, intravenous antibiotics should be continued until the patient is without fevers for at least 48 hours. If there is any evidence of necrosis, surgical debridement is required. Oral antibiotics should be continued for a 14-day course of therapy. Lesions can be quite painful and nonsteroidal anti-inflammatory drugs can offer both anti-inflammatory and analgesic benefits.

Outpatient Care

One of the most difficult aspects of treating vulvar lesions is the chronic nature of these diseases. The duration of treatment can range from 1 week to 6 months. Patients need to be closely monitored for new vulvar lesions that could exacerbate the original disease process. Finally, patients (along with their partners) should be counseled on the likelihood of remission and the chances of recurrences.

WHAT YOU NEED TO REMEMBER

- Using agents such as topical corticosteroids and warm compresses can help break the chronic itch-scratch cycle that aggravates vulvar lesions and inhibits the body's ability to heal.
- Good genital hygiene is critical to the successful resolution of most vulvar lesions.
- The most common solid vulvar lesion is a fibroma; Bartholin's gland enlargements are the most common cystic lesion of the vulva.
- If patients have ulceration, necrosis, or persistent pain/puritis, a punch biopsy is necessary to confirm the correct diagnosis.

SUGGESTED READINGS

American College of Obstetricians and Gynecologists. ACOG committee opinion number 345: vulvodynia. *Obstet Gynecol.* 2006;108:1049–1052.

American College of Obstetricians and Gynecologists. ACOG practice bulletin number 93: diagnosis and management of vulvar skin disorders. *Obstet Gynecol.* 2008;111:1243–1253.

Katz VL. Benign gynecologic lesions—vulva, vagina, cervix, uterus, oviduct, ovary. In: Katz VL, Lentz GM, Lobo RA, et al., eds. *Comprehensive Gynecology.* 5th ed. Philadelphia: Mosby Elsevier; 2007:419–473.

Pelvic Inflammatory Disease

THE PATIENT ENCOUNTER

A 22 year-old woman (G3P3), a new patient, arrives to the emergency department and you are called by the charge nurse to evaluate her. She presents with fever, lower abdominal pain, foul vaginal discharge, and general malaise.

OVERVIEW

The term *pelvic inflammatory disease* (PID) has been under close scrutiny in recent years because of the broad spectrum of anatomical areas possibly involved in every case, along with the polymicrobial nature of the process. The growing resistance of PID to common antibiotics and the rising incidence of cases among adolescents has made PID a major public health issue. This disease is closely related to infertility problems, and early detection of risk factors can prevent irreversible damage to the reproductive organs.

Definition

Pelvic inflammatory disease refers to the clinical syndrome that represents a spectrum of inflammatory and infectious disorders ascending from the vagina and cervix to the upper genital tract that involves the endometrium (endometritis), fallopian tubes (salpingitis), tubo-ovarian abscess, and pelvic peritoneum (peritonitis). Sometimes the infection can spread beyond the reproductive tract and cause pelvic abscess and generalized peritonitis, and it can affect other adjacent organs.

Pathophysiology

The presence of bacteria in the vaginal ecosystem and the risk factors associated with contracting a sexually transmitted disease in the genital tract, with its anatomic characteristics, explain the appearance of a PID. The connection between the vagina, the cervical canal, the endometrium, and the fallopian tubes provides an ascending path for the bacteria that cause this disease (1) (Fig. 17-1).

Epidemiology

During the 1990s, approximately 10% of women in their reproductive age reported having received treatment for a PID episode (2). This represents

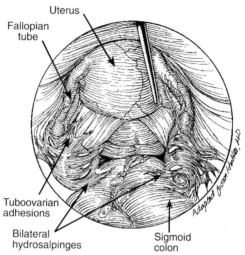

FIGURE 17-1: Sequelae of pelvic inflammatory disease.

only a small fraction of the possible cases that present every year. There is an underreporting of cases throughout the United States, mostly because of unsuspected cases or atypical clinical presentation. There are estimated to be between 9.5 and 14 cases per 1,000 fertile women, with the highest prevalence in women aged 15 to 24, ranging from 18 to 20 per 1,000. Each year, approximately 1 million cases of symptomatic PID occur in the United States (3). In 2002 in the United States, women 15 to 44 years of age made 200,000 initial visits to physicians offices for PID and approximately 66,000 were hospitalized for acute cases (4).

Etiology

Sexually transmitted organisms, such as *Neisseria gonorrhoeae* and *Chlamydia trachomatis*, are implicated in the etiology of PID (5). Table 17-1 lists the various organisms isolated from the vaginal flora. They can be categorized as sexually transmitted organisms, vaginal flora, and uncommon organisms. The clinical diagnosis of PID suggests that >80% of cases are infections caused by mixed organisms (6–9). Many risk factors are associated with PID. Age is inversely related to the incidence of PID. Sexually experienced teenagers have a threefold higher risk of being diagnosed with PID compared with women aged 25 to 29 years. Common risk factors associated with PID include the following:

- Young age at first intercourse
- Prior suicide attempt(s)
- Consumption of alcohol before sex

TABLE 17-1
Pathogen Organisms Frequently Implicated in Pelvic Inflammatory Disease Cases

STD-related organisms	*Neisseria gonorrhoeae, Chlamydia trachomatis*
Vaginal flora-related	*Enterobacteriaceae* spp., *Prevotella* spp., *Peptostreptococcus* spp., *Mycoplasma hominis, Streptococcus* spp., *Bacteroides* spp., *Fusobacterium* spp., *Gardnerella vaginalis, Escherichia coli, Streptococcus agalactiae, Streptococcus pneumoniae, Streptococcus pyogenes, Staphylococcus* spp., *Enterococcus* spp., *Pseudomonas* spp., *Mycobacterium tuberculosis, Neisseria meningitides, Actinomyces israelii.*
Other related organisms	*Haemophilus influenzae, Mycoplasma hominis,[a] Ureaplasma urealyticum[a]*

STD, sexually transmitted disease.
[a]Controversial involvement.

- Douching
- History of sexually transmitted disease (STD)
- Recent intrauterine device insertion
- Lack of barrier birth control method
- Substance abuse
- High-risk sexual partners
- Lower socioeconomic status
- Menses
- Cigarette smoking

ACUTE MANAGEMENT AND WORKUP

Pelvic inflammatory disease does not always present with classic symptoms. A systematic approach in cases with a high index of suspicion is critical for establishing the correct diagnosis.

The First 15 Minutes

Upon arrival to the emergency department or doctor's office, patients are usually in distress and feel sick. Always ensure the patient's initial health status; if critically ill, care should become a priority until the patient is stable.

Initial Assessment

The first thing to realize when facing a patient with a suspected PID is that symptoms can be mild but the degree of infection can be serious (10,11). The patient's vital signs at arrival will give you an idea of the general health status of your patient. A focused assessment should include the following:

1. *Ask the patient how she is feeling.* Evaluate whether she is alerted, oriented in time and space, and if she is able to respond correctly to your questions.
2. *Determine the patient's vital signs.* Is she febrile? Is she tachycardic? Is she breathing normally? What is her blood oxygen saturation? How is her blood pressure?
3. *Start evaluating her abdomen.* Listen for bowel movements with a stethoscope. Are they normal? Next, look for signs of lower abdominal signs of tenderness, or peritoneal irritability. Is lower abdominal pain present? Next, perform a pelvic exam; put the patient in the gynecologic position and insert a speculum. Look for cervical discharge or vaginal discharge. If present, take cultures and a Gram stain. Also perform a wet mount and a vaginal Ph measure. Next, do a bimanual exam, realizing that pain may be acutely triggered by your exam. Remember that you are looking for signs of tenderness in her cervix, uterus, or adnexa. Gently move her cervix and uterus sideways. Is pain present? Is it acute? Look for masses, enlarged ovaries, or uterine and/or general tenderness. Take note of every positive sign or symptom. Refer to Table 17-2 for minimum findings for diagnosis.
4. *Determine if the patient has intravenous (IV) access.* If not, start an IV access with normal saline solution or Ringer lactate. Start running it at 125 mL/hr.
5. *Obtain laboratory values.* While starting the IV access, take blood samples for laboratory tests. Refer to Table 17-2 for suggested laboratory tests to be ordered.
6. *Monitor the patient.* Keep the patient monitored at all times, until a final diagnosis is achieved.

Admission Criteria and Level of Care Criteria

The next step is to determine the patient's condition and severity of illness in the emergency department or doctor's office: Determine if the patient's condition is stable, fair, or critical.

Option 1: Stable Condition

Following the abdominal and pelvic exam, if mild signs are observed, vital signs and symptoms are stable or normal, and a wet mount reveals the

TABLE 17-2
Diagnostic Criteria for Pelvic Inflammatory Disease (PID)

Minimum findings	• Cervical motion tenderness • Adnexal and/or uterine tenderness • WBC observed on vaginal wet mount
Aggregated findings	• Oral temperature of 38.3°C (101°F) or higher • Abnormal cervical or vaginal mucopurulent discharge • Elevated erythrocyte sedimentation rate • Elevated C-reactive protein level
Additional oriented findings	• Laboratory documentation of infection with *Neisseria gonorrhoeae* or *Chlamydia trachomatis* • Positive histologic evidence of endometritis on endometrial biopsy • Radiologic abnormalities on vaginal ultrasound consistent with tubo-ovarian complex, fluid-filled tubes, free fluid on peritoneal cavity • Positive CT scan consistent with tubo-ovarian complex, fluid-filled tubes, free fluid on peritoneal cavity • Laparoscopic abnormalities consistent with PID • Leucocytosis 10,000 or more on CBC • Positive culdocentesis with purulent material • Purulent material in the peritoneal cavity obtained by laparoscopy

WBC, white blood count; CT, computed tomography; CBC, complete blood count.

absence of leucocytes and abundant bacteria consistent with a purulent discharge, considerations about ambulatory treatment may be considered. Remember to always rule out pregnancy.

Option 2: Fair Condition

Following the abdominal and pelvic exam, if mild-to-severe signs and symptoms are observed, vital signs are stable or normal, and a wet mount reveals the presence of abundant leucocytes and abundant bacteria consistent with a purulent discharge, ambulatory treatment should be started if the patient is reliable. Remember to always rule out pregnancy (12).

Option 3: Critical Condition

Following the abdominal and pelvic exam, if severe signs and symptoms are observed, vital signs are abnormal, fever is present with or without tachycardia and hypotension, a wet mount reveals the presence of abundant leucocytes and bacteria consistent with a purulent discharge, the white blood count (WBC) is elevated, and an ultrasound demonstrates a tubo-ovarian abscess, the patient should be immediately hospitalized and treated with IV antibiotics. Again, remember to always rule out pregnancy (12).

The First Few Hours

The first few hours are critical when the patient is hospitalized. The risk of sepsis or septic shock should be considered, and the patient should be kept under strict monitoring and surveillance. Follow-up on pending tests for confirmation of the severity of the disease is mandatory.

History

A good history will give you the diagnosis most of the time. Ask about the duration of symptom onset, temporal activities, and a history of prior STDs. Equally important is a history of any recent medications to treat the disease (either self-prescribed or under the supervision of another physician).

Physical Examination

The most important exam is the initial pelvic and abdominal examination. Serial exams over the next few hours are typically unnecessary except in the setting of an acute abdomen, in which severity could dictate surgical intervention.

Labs and Tests to Consider

A few simple tests can be performed to validate your clinical impression of PID. Laboratory findings, cultures, and imaging studies will help guide your decision about in-hospital versus outpatient treatment.

Key Diagnostic Labs and Tests

- Key diagnostic laboratory evaluation results that are indicative of PID include the following: WBC observed on vaginal wet mount
- Elevated erythrocyte sedimentation rate
- Elevated C-reactive protein level
- Laboratory documentation of infection with *N. gonorrhea* or *C. trachomatis*
- Histologic evidence of endometritis on endometrial biopsy
- Leukocytosis 10,000 or more on complete blood count (CBC)

In testing, remember to screen for other STDs.

Imaging

If the patient presents with an acute abdomen and appendicitis has not been excluded, a computed tomographic scan is the appropriate imaging exam.

Periodically, an adnexal mass is suspected during your initial pelvic exam, and a transvaginal ultrasound is best to exclude a tubo-ovarian abscess or a torsed ovary (13).

Treatment

Antibiotic therapy is generally given for 2 weeks. Mild cases of PID are treated on an outpatient basis using oral antibiotics (Table 17-3). The criteria for the hospitalization of patients with PID are any of the following:

- Surgical emergencies (e.g., appendicitis) cannot be excluded.
- The patient is pregnant.
- The patient does not respond clinically to oral antimicrobial therapy.
- The patient is unable to follow or tolerate an outpatient oral regimen.
- The patient has severe illness, nausea and vomiting, or high fever.

TABLE 17-3

Centers for Disease Control Recommendations for the Oral Treatment of Pelvic Inflammatory Disease

REGIMEN 1: RECOMMENDED ORAL REGIMEN
Ceftriaxone 250 mg intramuscularly in a single dose
PLUS
Doxycycline 100 mg orally twice a day for 14 days
with or without
Metronidazole 500 mg orally twice a day for 14 days

ALTERNATIVE 1:
Cefoxitin 2 g intramuscularly in a single dose, and **Probenecid**, 1 g orally administered concurrently in a single dose
plus
Doxycycline 100 mg orally twice a day for 14 days
with or without
Metronidazole 500 mg orally twice a day for 14 days

ALTERNATIVE 2:
Other parenteral third-generation **cephalosporin** (e.g., **ceftizoxime** or **cefotaxime**)
plus
Doxycycline 100 mg orally twice a day for 14 days
with or without
Metronidazole 500 mg orally twice a day for 14 days

- The patient has a tubo-ovarian abscess.
- There is no response to oral therapy after 72 hours.

CLINICAL PEARL

Young age and nulliparity are not necessarily indications for inpatient treatment of PID. The clinical response to outpatient therapy is similar in all age groups.

The CDC-approved regimens for parenteral therapy for PID are listed on Table 17-4.

EXTENDED IN-HOSPITAL MANAGEMENT

Patients who did not meet the criteria for outpatient management are treated with in-hospital parenteral antibiotics. Clinical improvement is

TABLE 17-4

Centers for Disease Control Recommendations for the Parenteral Treatment of Pelvic Inflammatory Disease

RECOMMENDED PARENTERAL REGIMEN A
Cefotetan 2 g intravenously every 12 hours
or
Cefoxitin 2 g intravenously every 6 hours
plus
Doxycycline 100 mg orally or intravenously every 12 hours

RECOMMMENDED PARENTERAL REGIMEN B
Clindamycin 900 mg intravenously every 8 hours
plus
Gentamicin loading dose intravenously or intramuscularly (2 mg/kg of body weight), followed by a maintenance dose (1.5 mg/kg) every 8 hours. Single daily dosing may be substituted.

ALTERNATIVE PARENTERAL REGIMENS
Ampicillin/Sulbactam 3 g intravenously every 6 hours
plus
Doxycycline 100 mg orally or intravenously every 12 hours

monitored using both subjective and objective data. Subjectively, decreasing discomfort with pelvic exams and pain scores are reassuring signs of improvement. Objectively, a downward trending WBC and temperature curve can help gauge when a patient is ready for discharge. During the hospitalization, adequate pain control is essential. Finally, a thorough discussion regarding safe sex practices and contraception should be initiated during this hospitalization.

DISPOSITION

Discharge Goals

Goals for discharge are the following:

- Vital signs demonstrate that the patient is stable.
- The CBC leucocytes count is near normal.
- General symptoms have disappeared.
- The patient is able to tolerate oral treatment.

Outpatient Care

Pelvic rest for at least 2 weeks is prudent while the patient is completing her complete course of antibiotics. A follow-up visit in 1 to 2 weeks is required for the evaluation of the clinical resolution of symptoms. Time should be spent with the patient explaining the possible sequelae of the disease, which is important in follow-up care, especially for the early detection of recurrences (14).The list of possible sequelae of PID is provided in Table 17-5.

TABLE 17-5
Potential Sequelae of Pelvic Inflammatory Disease (PID)

Potential Sequelae in General	Potential Sequelae of Fertility

• TOA
• Recurrent PID
• Chronic or recurrent abdominal pain or pelvic pain
• Dyspareunia
• Dysmenorrhea
• Adhesive disease
• Ectopic pregnancy
	• Infertility, risk after PID
	  • 1st episode, 8 to 13%
	  • 2nd episode, 20 to 35%
	  • 3rd episode, 40 to 75%
	• If true TOA is present, only 7 to 14% patients will conceive after treatment

TOA, tubo-ovarian abscess.

CLINICAL PEARL

Some experts recommend rescreening for gonorrhea and chlamydia 4 to 6 weeks after treatment if the organisms were documented as the source of infection to confirm a test of cure.

WHAT YOU NEED TO REMEMBER

- Pelvic inflammatory disease is a frequently encountered disease, with approximately 1 million cases per year in the United States.
- The main diagnostic clinical features include pelvic pain; tenderness in the cervix, uterus, or adnexa during the pelvic exam; fever; and leukocytosis on the wet mount or CBC.
- Lab work and radiology workup are suggested for an accurate definition of the severity of disease.
- Follow-up should be arranged 2 weeks after treatment and/or discharge.

REFERENCES

1. Westrom L, Wolner-Hanssen P. Pathogenesis of pelvic inflammatory disease. *Genitourin Med.* 1993;69:9–17.
2. Aral SO, Mosher WD, Cates W. Self-reported pelvic inflammatory disease in the United States, 1998. *JAMA.* 1991;266:2570–2573.
3. Mandell GL, Bennett JE, Dolin R. *Principles and Practice of Infectious Diseases.* 6th ed, New York: Elsevier Churchill Livingstone; 2006:1378–1380.
4. Kasper DL, Braunwald E, Fauci AS, et al. *Harrison's Principles of Internal Medicine.* 16th ed. New York: McGraw Hill; 2006:769–771.
5. Mardh P-A, Moller BR, Paavonen J. Chlamydial infection of the female genital tract with emphasis on pelvic inflammatory disease: a review of Scandinavian studies. *Sex Transm Dis.* 1981;8:140–155.
6. Eschenbach DA, Buchanan TM, Pollock HM, et al. Polymicrobial etiology of acute pelvic inflammatory disease. *N Engl J Med.* 1975;293:166–171.
7. Cunningham FG, Hauth JC, Gilstrap LC, et al. The bacterial pathogenesis of acute pelvic inflammatory disease. *Obstet Gynecol.* 1978;52:161–164.
8. Chow WC, Malkasian KL, Marshall JR, et al. The bacteriology of acute pelvic inflammatory disease: value cul-de-sac cultures and relative importance of gonococci and other aerobic and anaerobic bacteria. *Am J Obstet Gynecol.* 1975;122:876–879.
9. Monif GRG, Welkos SL, Baer H, et al. Cul-de-sac isolates from patients with endometritis-salpingitis-peritonitis and gonococcal endocervicitis. *Am J Obstet Gynecol.* 1976;126:158–161.

10. Washington AE, Aral SO, Wolner-Hanssen P, et al. Assessing risk for pelvic inflammatory disease and its sequelae. *JAMA*. 1991;266:2581–2586.
11. Ness RB, Keder LM, Soper DE, et al. Oral contraception and the recognition of endometritis. *Am J Obstet Gynecol*. 1997;176:580–585.
12. Faro S, Soper D. Pelvic inflammatory disease. In: *Infectious Diseases in Women*. New York: McGraw Hill; 2002:287–299.
13. Patten RM, Vincent LM, Wolner-Hanssen P, et al. Pelvic inflammatory disease: endovaginal sonography with laparoscopic correlation. *J Ultrasound Med*. 1990;9:681–689.
14. Safrin S, Schachter J, Dahrouge D, et al. Long-term sequelae of acute pelvic inflammatory disease: a retrospective cohort study. *Am J Obstet Gynecol*. 1992; 166:1300–1305.

SUGGESTED READINGS

Centers for Disease Control. Sexually Transmitted Diseases Treatment Guidelines, 2006. *MMWR*. 2006;55(RR-11):1–94.
Centers for Disease Control. MMWR update to CDCs sexually transmitted diseases treatment guidelines, 2006: fluoroquinolones no longer recommended for treatment of gonococcal infections. *MMWR*. 2007;56(14);332–336.
Moniff G, Baker D. *Infectious Diseases in Obstetrics and Gynecology*. 5th ed. Nashville, TN: Parthenon Publishing; 2004.

Abnormal Uterine Bleeding

A 45-year-old patient (G4P4) presents to your office with the complaint that she has been "bleeding off and on, but mostly on" for 6 weeks. She has always had heavy flow, but her periods have become more irregular and heavier over time, and they have caused her a great deal of inconvenience. At times she soaks through a pad in <1 hour. Today she continues to bleed and she complains that she is feeling weak and light-headed.

OVERVIEW

Definition

Abnormal uterine bleeding (AUB) is one of the most common presenting conditions in gynecology. Normal menstrual bleeding lasts between 2 days and 7 days, and abnormal bleeding can mean excessive bleeding or bleeding outside the normal menstrual cycle. This includes the following:

- Menorrhagia (>80 mL, or more practically, soaking through more than about 1 pad per hour, or >30 pads per cycle)
- Oligomenorrhea (infrequent periods)
- Polymenorrhea (frequent periods)
- Metrorrhagia (bleeding between regular cycles)
- Menometrorrhagia (irregular and heavy bleeding)

Pathophysiology

Causes of abnormal bleeding can be divided into two categories: organic and dysfunctional. Organic causes include systemic and reproductive tract etiologies (Table 18-1 presents a list of organic causes). Leiomyomas, or fibroids, are a common reproductive tract cause of abnormal uterine bleeding. These pseudoencapsulated benign tumors of smooth muscle and fibrous connective tissue are found in the myometrium and can cause heavy or intermenstrual bleeding, especially if the fibroid is large or submucosal.

Dysfunctional endocrinologic bleeding includes anovulatory and ovulatory causes. Endometrial hyperplasia results from high estrogen levels along with insufficient progesterone. In a premenopausal woman, anovulation is one of the most common causes of AUB. In the absence of ovulation,

TABLE 18-1
Organic Etiologies of Abnormal Uterine Bleeding

Systemic	Reproductive Tract

• Von Willebrand disease
• Prothrombin deficiency
• Platelet deficiency
  • Leukemia
  • Sepsis
  • Idiopathic thrombocytopenic purpura
  • Hypersplenia
• Coagulopathies
• Hypothyroidism
• Cirrhosis
• Renal failure
	• Pregnancy accidents
	  • Threatened abortion
	  • Missed abortion
	  • Incomplete abortion
	  • Ectopic pregnancy
	• Trophoblastic disease
	• Endometrial cancer
	• Cervical cancer
	• Estrogen-producing tumor
	• Endometritis
	• Endometriosis
	• Submucosal myomas
	• Endometrial polyps
	• Adenomyosis
	• Cervical lesion or erosion
	• Cervicitis
	• Intrauterine device

no progesterone is produced to stabilize the estrogen-induced endometrial proliferation. Continuous growth without progesterone causes buildup of the uterine lining over time and sporadic blood loss. Irregular ovulation is most common in adolescence, due to an immature hypothalamic pituitary axis, and in perimenopause, due to disturbed cyclic hormone production. Abnormal ovulatory bleeding during the reproductive years is thought to be due to idiopathic abnormal prostaglandin metabolism related to an imbalance in the ratio of vasoconstrictive prostaglandin $F_2\alpha$ and vasodilating prostaglandin E.

Epidemiology

Approximately 10% of healthy women have heavy uterine bleeding—it is one of the most common complaints women have when they visit their gynecologist (1). Approximately 13% of cases of AUD in adolescents who present with heavy vaginal bleeding since the onset of menses are due to von Willebrand deficiency. Finally, in women older than age 35, uterine fibroids account for 25% of the cases (2).

Etiology

The risk of developing endometrial hyperplasia is correlated with unopposed estrogen exposure and is related to obesity, diabetes, chronic anovulation, or estrogen therapy. The incidence increases with each decade during the reproductive years and is highest in the perimenopausal age group.

ACUTE MANAGEMENT AND WORKUP

Hemodynamic stability is the primary focus of managing a patient with acute, heavy menses.

The First 15 Minutes

The first step in management is to assess the patient's hemodynamic state and to determine the need for intravenous fluid resuscitation or transfusion. Check the patient's vital signs for tachycardia, orthostatic hypotension, and tachypnea, and ensure that the patient is alert and oriented.

Initial Assessment

Some patients with abnormal bleeding may present to the emergency department in a critical hemorrhagic state, but most are hemodynamically stable enough to walk in for a scheduled office visit. However, even an ambulatory patient may have a critically low hemoglobin level. She may appear pale and complain of weakness, light-headedness, fatigue, or shortness of breath. Adolescent patients, who, in addition, may not be alarmed at their bleeding pattern because they do not recognize it as irregular, are especially able to tolerate anemia and compensate very well until they reach a critical point. Thus, it is vital to check a stat hemoglobin level in your initial assessment, as well as to check a urine pregnancy test. Ectopic pregnancies must be excluded in the face of hemorrhagic shock and a positive pregnancy test.

Admission Criteria and Level of Care Criteria

Acute care may be necessary in the instance of severe acute blood loss. Consider admission of the patient with a hemoglobin level of 7 g/dL or less, depending on age, hemodynamic stability, and the presence of other medical conditions.

The First few Hours

Dangerously heavy uterine bleeding can be managed with pharmacologic-dose estrogen therapy to stabilize the endometrial lining and stop acute bleeding. Excessive blood loss should be replaced with crystalline fluids or blood transfusion. If there is no response to estrogen therapy within 24 hours, an emergency dilatation and curettage (D&C) is appropriate to stop bleeding.

History

A full history should be obtained with focus on a description of the menstrual bleeding and its pattern. Questions to ask the patient include the following:

- How many days does it last?
- How many days are there between bleeds?
- How much blood is lost in pads per hour or total pads per cycle?
- How long has it been irregular?
- How does this impact the patient's quality of life?
- Are there associated symptoms of abdominal pain, vaginal discharge, cramping, or fever?

Disorders of pregnancy are also an important cause of abnormal bleeding in any woman who is not menopausal. In the first trimester, bleeding can be an early sign of miscarriage or even of an ectopic pregnancy (especially if the patient has had surgical sterilization and has one-sided pain). Later in pregnancy, bleeding can be from placental problems. You should always confirm that your patient's pregnancy test is negative.

You should also ask if there is a family history of endometrial hyperplasia or carcinoma. Bleeding disorders, such as Von Willebrand disease, thrombocytopenia, or another coagulopathy, can be screened for by asking if the patient or anyone in the family bleeds easily. A hypothalamic etiology may be suggested by a history of increased stress, an eating disorder, or excessive exercise. The presence of an intrauterine device can cause abnormal bleeding, and oral contraceptives (especially low-estrogen or progestin-only preparations) may cause breakthrough bleeding due to the endometrium adjusting to a thinner state. Hirsutism or signs of excess androgen may suggest polycystic ovary syndrome. Postcoital bleeding may point to endometritis and cervicitis as the source of bleeding. You can also determine the patent's ovulatory status based on premenstrual symptoms of breast tenderness, weight gain, abdominal cramping, and mood swings.

Physical Examination

A pelvic exam is necessary, even if patient is actively bleeding, to identify infection, uterine fibroids, polyps, adnexal masses, internal or external trauma, or an alternate source (such as the urethra or rectum) as the cause of the bleeding (Fig. 18-1). You can assess the amount of bleeding the patient is having based on the amount of blood or clots in vaginal vault, as well as identify active bleeding from the cervix. Polyps or cervical masses may be visible or palpable, and a presumptive diagnosis of fibroids can be made by an abdominal and pelvic exam that reveals firm, nontender, smooth, and mobile nodules or masses arising from the uterus.

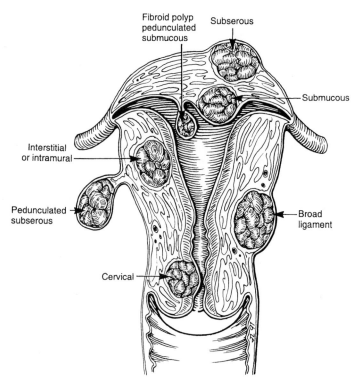

FIGURE 18-1: Common types of uterine fibroids.

Labs and Tests to Consider

Laboratory evaluations include key blood tests, such as complete blood count (CBC), beta-human chorionic gonadotropin (β-hCG), and thyroid function testing. Key imaging includes transvaginal ultrasound, saline sono-histography, and hysteroscopy.

Key Diagnostic Labs and Tests

After a stat CBC and qualitative β-hCG to rule out pregnancy or ectopic pregnancy, thyroid function testing is important for the assessment of anovulatory bleeding. In addition, prolactin levels should be checked in a patient with oligomenorrhea; platelet function analysis is indicated for severe menorrhagia or other signs of coagulopathy.

Because cervical cancer commonly presents with abnormal bleeding, every patient should have a Pap smear performed as soon as possible if she has not had one in the last year. Any suspicious lesions found on physical exam should be biopsied, and cervical smears for should be sent for cytology and culture study.

Imaging

Transvaginal ultrasound can be very useful to evaluate for a structural problem (fibroids, polyp, adnexal mass), to rule out an intrauterine or ectopic pregnancy, and to evaluate endometrial thickness.

CLINICAL PEARL

Endometrial biopsies should be considered in women at high risk for developing hyperplasia: age >35, prolonged unopposed estrogen exposure, obesity, or polycystic ovary syndrome.

Because the incidence of endometrial hyperplasia and malignancy rises in the perimenopausal and postmenopausal years, there should be a lower threshold for endometrial assessment.

Sonohistogram with saline infusion into the uterus may help to differentiate between an endometrial polyp and submucous myomas. Hysteroscopy has the advantage of having the ability to remove a polyp if one is found. Computed tomography scans are obtained to look for evidence of metastatic disease if the provider has a high index of suspicion for gynecologic cancer.

Treatment

Most patients with AUB can be managed conservatively with medical treatment (Table 18-2). In anovulatory bleeding, the goal of treatment is to minimize blood loss, regulate cycles, and prevent the complications of unopposed chronic estrogen. Women younger than age 45 with no risk factors for endometrial cancer can be started on a low-dose oral contraceptive pill (OCP) to regulate bleeding. These pills are also very useful in adolescents to regulate cyclic bleeding until the hypothalamic-pituitary feedback system matures.

In patients with contraindications to estrogen therapy or with less significant bleeding, cyclic progesterone can be used. Contraindications to estrogen therapy include the following:

- Prior thrombotic event
- Cigarette smoking
- Hypercoagulable states, such as factor V Leiden
- Rheumatoid disease
- Liver disease
- Estrogen-responsive cancer

Progesterone stimulates conversion of proliferative to organized secretory endometrium, and then is withdrawn to cause regular bleeding. In addition to oral dosing, progestins can be given in the form of an intrauterine

TABLE 18-2
Summary of Medical Treatments for Abnormal Uterine Bleeding

Use	Medication	Dosage	Mechanism
Stop acute hemorrhagic bleeding	Estrogen	25 mg IV every 6 hours for 24 hours or 10 mg/day in divided into 4 doses or 4 × 50 mcg OCPs at one time	Rapid endometrial growth stabilizes lining to stop acute bleeding.
	NSAIDs	Standard dosage monthly while menstruating	Modulates vasodilating prostaglandins to slow bleeding for 24 hours
Anovulatory bleeding	Combination OCP	Many different combinations	Regulates cyclic bleeding with timed withdrawal bleeds
	Progesterone (medroxyprogesterone) Marina IUD	10 mg for 10 days per month	Organizes endometrial growth and allows for organized sloth with withdrawal. Also opposes estrogen effect.

	Clomiphene Citrate	50 mg PO Daily for 5 days	Antiestrogen for ovulation induction in women who desire fertility.
	NSAIDs	Standard dosage monthly while menstruating	Decrease heaviness and flow during menstruation
Oligomenorrhea	Monophasic OCP	TID for 5–7 days, then daily dosing for 3 weeks, followed by a withdrawal bleed. A combination OCP is used thereafter.	Induces withdrawal bleed if none in last 6 weeks; regulates cycle thereafter.
Fibroids	Progesterone (norethindrone) or	10 mg daily	
	medroxyprogesterone (Depo-Provera)	200 mg IM once monthly	
	Combination OCP	Many different combinations	Regulates cyclic bleeding with timed withdrawal bleeds

(continued)

TABLE 18-2

Summary of Medical Treatments for Abnormal Uterine Bleeding (Continued)

Use	Medication	Dosage	Mechanism
Bleeding refractory to other medical treatment	Leuprolide (Lupron or Lupron Depot)	0.5–1.0 mg/day or 3.75–7.5 mg/month	GnRH agonists
	Nafarelin (Synarel)	Intranasal 200 mcg BID	
	Goserelin (Zoladex)	Implant 3.6 mg SC every 4 weeks for 6 months	

IV, intravenously; OCP, oral contraceptive pill; NSAID, nonsteroidal anti-inflammatory drug; IUD, intrauterine device; PO, orally; TID, three times a day; IM, intramuscularly; GnRH, gonadotropin-releasing hormone; BID, two times a day; SC, subcutaneously.

device and continuously delivered directly to the uterine cavity to decrease menstrual flow, often resulting in amenorrhea. In patients who desire fertility, clomiphene citrate can be used for ovulation induction.

With oligomenorrhea due to hypothalamic-pituitary dysfunction, it is also important to maintain adequate estrogen to support bone health. An OCP is appropriate treatment here, as well as for oligomenorrhea due to anovulation.

Patients with fibroids that cause minimal symptoms can be managed conservatively with iron replacement, analgesics, or progestins to reduce the amount of bleeding. Progesterone therapy does not reduce the size of the fibroid.

Luteinizing hormone and follicle-stimulating hormone suppressants or gonadotropin-releasing hormone agonists can be used for bleeding refractory to other treatment. These agents create an abrupt artificial menopause secondary to decreased gonadotropins, causing cessation of bleeding and the shrinkage of fibroids due to a lack of estrogen. This therapy is not recommended for >6 months but may be used as an adjunct in preparation for surgery in the perimenopausal patient. Calcium supplementation (1,000–1,500 mg/day) should be added to this regimen to maintain the bones in this hypoestrogenic state.

In addition, the bleeding patient should be given an iron supplement as well as antiemetics if the patient's regimen requires more than one OCP pill per day. A preliminary Pap smear, an endometrial biopsy, or a D&C are also important, especially in older patients, to rule out premalignant pathology.

When medical management fails, more invasive interventions may be necessary. A D&C can stop acute bleeding, and also aids in ruling out cervical or uterine carcinomas. If hyperplasia with atypia is found in the D&C, you should suspect a nearby adenocarcinoma. Hysteroscopic endometrial ablation is an effective treatment for hypermenorrhea, and myolysis of fibroids can be accomplished by needle cautery, laser, cryotherapy, or thermal balloon. Finally, lysis of uterine adhesions, excision of fibroids, uterine artery embolization, or total abdominal hysterectomy (especially if future fertility is not desired) are the most invasive methods to cease uterine bleeding. Laparoscopy may also be useful in complex cases and in ruling out other pelvic pathology.

EXTENDED IN-HOSPITAL MANAGEMENT

There are few cases severe enough to require a hysterectomy, but emergency surgery and hospitalization may be necessary for severe bleeding, or when medical treatment fails. Following laparotomy, the patient should be monitored in the hospital for 2 to 4 days followed by limited activity and pelvic rest (including no sexual intercourse) for 1 month. Hysteroscopic or laparoscopic procedures require limited activity for 24 hours and pelvic rest for 2 weeks. While recovering in the hospital, the patient's hematocrit level should be followed and her hemodynamic stability monitored.

DISPOSITION

Discharge Goals

The patient may be released from inpatient care when she is hemodynamically stable and the uterine bleeding is controlled by medical or surgical therapy.

Outpatient Care

Follow-up care with regular office visits is important to monitor symptoms every 8 to 12 weeks, and, if necessary, to reassess any pathology that was found.

Small, asymptomatic fibroids can be managed conservatively with pelvic examinations and ultrasonography at 3- to 6-month intervals, as long as they remain a stable size. They should regress after menopause.

 WHAT YOU NEED TO REMEMBER

- The patient with abnormal uterine bleeding should have a CBC, β-hCG, and thyrotropin levels checked.
- Endometrial biopsy should be obtained in patients over age 35 or with a history of prolonged estrogen exposure.
- If vaginal bleeding begins 6 or more months after the cessation of menstruation, then you must assume that it is cancer-related until it is ruled out.

REFERENCES

1. Katz VL, Gershenson DM, Lobo RA, et al., eds. *Comprehensive Gynecology.* 5th ed. Philadelphia: Mosby; 2007.
2. Fazio SB, Ship AN. Abnormal uterine bleeding. *S Med J.* 2007;100:376–382.

SUGGESTED READINGS

American College of Obstetricians and Gynecologists. ACOG practice bulletin number 14: management of anovulatory bleeding. (March 2000). Available at: www.acog.org/publications/educational-bulletins/pb014.cfm. Accessed July 30, 2008.

American College of Obstetricians and Gynecologists. ACOG practice bulletin 16: alternatives to hysterectomy and management of leiomyomas. *Obstet Gynecol.* 2008;112:201–207.

Ely JW, Kennedy CM, Clark EC, et al. Abnormal uterine bleeding: a management algorithm. *J Am Board Fam Med.* 2006;19:590–602.

Telner DE, Jakubovicz D. Approach to diagnosis and management of abnormal uterine bleeding. Clinical Review Series on Women's Health. *Can Fam Physician.* 2007;53:58–64.

Adnexal Masses

THE PATIENT ENCOUNTER

You are working in the emergency department when a 26-year-old woman (G1P1) presents, complaining of severe left lower quadrant pain that began suddenly 3 hours ago. The patient also reports nausea and vomiting since the onset of the pain. When you first see the patient, she is writhing in obvious, severe pain, and she has peritoneal signs upon examination. A pelvic ultrasound exam shows a 5-cm left adnexal mass with no blood flow to the left ovary.

OVERVIEW

Definition

Adnexa refers to the structures adjoining the uterus, including the fallopian tubes, the ovaries, and also the blood vessels, ligaments, and connective tissues (1). Adnexal masses may be symptomatic, as described in the case presented here, or may be found incidentally on examination or in imaging studies. Some adnexal masses are completely benign and require no treatment, others can present as surgical emergencies, and others present be life-threatening malignancies that need immediate attention.

Pathophysiology

Adnexal masses may be of gynecologic or nongynecologic origin, as outlined in Table 19-1. There are certain clinical characteristics that we can use to help differentiate between benign and malignant masses (Table 19-2).

Epidemiology

Adnexal masses can be found in females of all ages, from fetuses to postmenopausal women. The prevalence of reported ranges depends on the population studied and the methods used for diagnosis. One study of 335 asymptomatic women ages 25 to 40 showed a point prevalence of an adnexal mass by ultrasound examination to be 7.8% (1).

Etiology

There are many causes of adnexal masses, and they vary greatly depending on the age group.

TABLE 19-1
Classification of Adnexal Masses

Masses of Gynecologic Origin	Masses of Nongynecologic Origin
Ovarian follicular cyst	Appendiceal abscess
Corpus luteum cyst	Diverticulosis
Theca-lutein cyst	Adhesions of bowel and omentum
Luteoma of pregnancy	Peritoneal cyst
Polycystic ovaries	Feces in rectosigmoid
Inflammatory cyst	Urine in bladder
Ectopic pregnancy	Pelvic kidney
Congenital abnormality	Urachal cyst
Embryologic remnant	Anterior sacral meningocele
Pyosalpinx	Sigmoid carcinoma
Hydrosalpinx	Cecum carcinoma
Bladder	Retroperitoneal neoplasm
Leiomyomata	Presacral teratoma
Paraovarian cyst	
Ovarian neoplasm	
Endometrial neoplasm	
Tubal neoplasm	

Premenarche

The causes of adnexal masses during premenarche include the following (2):

- *Follicular cysts* are found in infants and occur by maternal hormone stimulation of the fetal ovaries. They generally regress spontaneously in the first few months of life.
- *Benign ovarian tumors* in this age group are most often mature teratomas, also known as dermoids. They may contain elements of all three germ layers, including teeth, hair, and sebum.
- *Malignant ovarian tumors* include dysgerminomas, immature teratomas, endodermal sinus tumors, and embryonal carcinomas.
- *Nongynecologic causes* include Wilms tumor, neuroblastoma, and gastrointestinal tumors.

TABLE 19-2
Clinical Findings that Suggest a Benign or Malignant Adnexal Mass

Benign Masses	Malignant Masses
Unilateral	Bilateral
Cystic	Solid
Mobile	Fixed
Smooth	Irregular
No ascites	Ascites
Slow growth	Rapid growth
Adolescent patient	Postmenopausal patient

Menarche

The causes of adnexal masses during menarche include the following:

- *Functional cysts* are the *most common by far*. They are produced by the ovary during each menstrual cycle. They are normally 3- to 10-cm simple cysts (2).
- *Paratubal and paraovarian cysts* are also quite common. They arise from mesonephric structures. They are thin-walled and benign (2).
- *Benign ovarian tumors*
  - *Mature teratomas (dermoids)* are the most common benign ovarian tumor in this age group as well. They may be up to 10 cm in size. They also may cause adnexal torsion and present as an acute abdomen. Teeth and bone may be detectable in the mass by ultrasound (2)
  - *Serous and mucinous cystadenomas* are thin-walled unilocular or multilocular masses that may range from 5 cm to >20 cm in size. Mucinous cystadenomas are usually larger and are less likely to be bilateral than serous cystadenomas (3).
  - *Endometriomas* are caused by the growth of endometrial tissue outside the uterus. Patients often complain of dysmenorrhea, dyspareunia, and chronic pelvic pain (3).
- *Malignant ovarian tumors* of all types must be on the differential in this age group (see the following section, *Postmenopause*, for details).
- *Pregnancy-related adnexal masses*
  - *Ectopic pregnancy* must be number one on the list of differential diagnoses in women with a positive pregnancy test and an adnexal mass. This can be a surgical emergency.

- *Theca-lutein cysts* are luteinized follicle cysts that arise from overstimulation of the ovary from high levels of human chorionic gonadotropin (hCG) in pregnancy (3). They are usually bilateral, multiseptated cystic masses. They are often seen in patients with trophoblastic disease or multiple gestations due to the higher levels of hCG, but also may be seen in normal pregnancy (3).
- *Corpus luteum of pregnancy* is found in all early intrauterine pregnancies and is usually smaller than 3 cm in size. It produces progesterone to support the pregnancy in the first 7 to 10 weeks of gestation (4).
- *Luteomas* represent an exaggerated luteinization reaction of the normal ovary in pregnancy. They are typically a solid, complex-appearing unilateral or bilateral mass on ultrasound. They may cause maternal virilization (4).
- *Leiomyomas (fibroids)* are composed of smooth muscle cells and are benign. They are found in as many as 30% of women of reproductive age (2). *Tubo-ovarian abscesses* are often accompanied by fever and other systemic signs of infection.
- *Polycystic ovary syndrome* is a condition in which the ovaries appear multicystic on ultrasound. Clinical features include obesity, anovulation, infertility, and hirsutism (1).

Postmenopause

Although all of the previously described benign causes of adnexal masses still may be found in this age group, the chance of an adnexal mass being malignant increases with age. An adnexal mass in a postmenopausal woman should be considered malignant until proven otherwise. The types of malignant ovarian tumors are the following:
- Epithelial ovarian cancer (85%–90%)
  - The median age of diagnosis is 61 years.
  - A woman has a 1-in-56 lifetime risk of developing ovarian cancer.
  - Risk factors: Low parity, genetic predisposition (*BRCA1* or *BRCA2*)
  - Protective factors: Multiparity, oral contraceptive use, breast-feeding, and chronic anovulation
  - Signs and symptoms: Ovarian cancer is often asymptomatic until the late stages. Vague complaints, such as abdominal discomfort, bloating, and early satiety, are often overlooked, making an early diagnosis difficult.
  - 75% of patients present with stage III-IV disease.
  - Tumor marker: CA-125
  - Treatment: Complete surgical staging and maximal tumor cytoreduction, followed by chemotherapy with six cycles of carboplatin and paclitaxel (5).
- Germ cell tumors (5%–7%)

- Dysgerminoma: This is the most common type (50%). The median age of diagnosis is 17 years. Lactate dehydrogenase is a useful tumor marker. The overall survival rate is 85%.
- Endodermal sinus tumor: This is the second most common type. The median age of diagnosis is 19 years. The tumor marker is alpha-fetoprotein.
- Other types: Immature teratomas, embryonal carcinomas, choriocar-cinoma.
- Treatment: If a woman desires to preserve fertility, then unilateral oophorectomy is appropriate management; otherwise, complete surgical staging should be performed (5).
- Sex cord stromal tumors (5%–7%)
  - Granulosa cell tumors: These are the most common type (70%). Inhibin A and B are tumor markers.
  - Sertoli-Leydig tumors: These tumors are rare. They often present as signs of virilization in young, reproductive-age women.
  - Treatment: This is the same as for germ cell tumors. These are low-grade malignancy tumors that rarely recur (5).

ACUTE MANAGEMENT AND WORKUP
The First 15 Minutes
The most important question to answer in the first 15 minutes is whether or not your patient requires emergent surgical intervention. Severe pain and/or hemodynamic instability are the two primary reasons for proceeding with surgery.

Initial Assessment
One of the most critical skills to acquire as a physician is the ability to determine who is sick and who is not sick. You must first determine the acuity of the patient's condition:

1. *Determine the patient's mental status.* Is the patient alert and able to answer questions? In the first few minutes, you want to gather a brief, pertinent history that will allow you to form a differential diagnosis. If the patient is unresponsive or obtunded, she is clearly sick and needs immediate care.
2. *Check the patient's vital signs.* If the patient is hypotensive or tachycardic, this indicates hemodynamic instability that requires immediate intervention. Fever should raise suspicion for infection, which also requires timely treatment to avoid sepsis.
3. *Examine the patient.* In the first few minutes, your job is to determine if the patient requires emergent surgical intervention. Does the patient have evidence of an acute abdomen, such as peritoneal signs? Highest on the list of differential diagnoses in a patient with an adnexal mass and an

acute abdomen are adnexal torsion, ruptured tubo-ovarian abscess, which causes diffuse peritonitis, or a ruptured ectopic pregnancy. In all cases, the patient will needed immediate surgical exploration.

Admission Criteria and Level of Care Criteria

If the patient does not require immediate surgical intervention for her adnexal mass, outpatient management is generally accepted. In cases in which a patient has a somewhat concerning exam but no need for emergent surgical intervention, an admission for observation with serial exams may be appropriate in order to ensure that the patient's condition does not worsen acutely. Asymptomatic adnexal masses that meet criteria for surgical removal can be scheduled for surgery on an outpatient basis and generally do not require immediate hospitalization.

The First Few Hours

Once you have established that the patient is stable, you will need to perform a thorough workup to determine the diagnosis as well as the management and treatment that the patient will require.

History

After any emergent issues have been addressed, obtain a thorough history. Is the patient having pain? If so, find out how long she has been having pain. Has there been an acute change in her pain, which would be more concerning for torsion, or is this a dull, chronic type of pain that is more like a stable mass that has been present for some time? Very severe pain earlier in the presentation that has since resolved may be falsely reassuring. This could indicate an adnexal torsion that has led to an ischemic ovary that is no longer painful because of nerve death, so don't be fooled. Acute onset of nausea and vomiting should raise your suspicion for torsion. Ask about subtle symptoms that are so frequently overlooked, such as early satiety, or increasing abdominal girth, which may indicate malignancy. Also find out if breast or ovarian cancer runs in the family as this could also raise your suspicion for malignancy.

Physical Examination

A complete physical exam is necessary in evaluating all patients. The aspects to focus on pertaining to adnexal masses are an abdominal exam, and a bimanual and rectovaginal exam.

Abdominal Examination

First, you must determine if the patient has signs of an acute abdomen, such as rebound tenderness, muscular rigidity, or hypoactive bowel signs. It is also important to palpate for masses because pelvic masses can grow to a size that is easily palpable abdominally. Remember to look for a fluid wave, or other signs of ascites, that would be concerning for malignancy.

Bimanual and Rectovaginal Examination

This exam should be performed to evaluate the size, location, mobility, and consistency of an adnexal mass. Normal ovaries in a postmenopausal woman should be nonpalpable, so a palpable mass in a postmenopausal woman should raise concern for malignancy. An immobile mass in a premenopausal woman could signify endometriosis, but this finding in a postmenopausal woman is also concerning for malignancy. Tenderness of the adnexa often represents infection, but may also be seen with any adnexal mass (6).

Labs and Tests to Consider

Laboratory tests and other tests in a patient with an adnexal mass should be ordered according to the patient's clinical presentation.

Key Diagnostic Labs and Tests

If the patient presents with nausea, vomiting, and fever, it is appropriate to order laboratory workups to fully evaluate these symptoms. These tests include a complete blood work with differential, electrolytes, and liver function tests. If the patient presents with an asymptomatic adnexal mass, tumor markers may be indicated. CA-125 is not a useful diagnostic or screening test for ovarian cancer as it is neither sensitive nor specific for the disease. However, it is appropriate to order a CA-125 evaluation in a premenopausal woman with an adnexal mass that is suspicious by ultrasound, or in any postmenopausal woman with an adnexal mass. Although the CA-125 level is not diagnostic, it may be helpful as a baseline measurement to help guide treatment if the patient is found to have ovarian cancer. Other tumor markers, such as alpha-fetoprotein, lactate dehydrogenase, or hCG, may be drawn if suspicion for germ cell tumors is high based on the clinical picture, such as the presence of a solid adnexal mass in a premenarchal or adolescent patient (6).

Imaging

The best way to image the pelvis for adnexal masses is with ultrasound. Transabdominal and transvaginal ultrasound should be performed to best assess both abdominal and pelvic processes. In a patient with suspected adnexal torsion, Doppler can be used to assess blood flow to the ovary.

CLINICAL PEARL

Although reduced or absent blood flow to the ovary is suggestive of adnexal torsion, the diagnosis cannot be made solely on this finding. In addition, the presence of blood flow in the adnexa cannot be used to exclude the diagnosis of torsion, as some collateral blood flow may be preserved even in cases of clinically significant adnexal torsion.

There are also some sonographic characteristics have been associated with greater likelihood of malignancy:

- Solid component that is not hyperechoic and is often nodular or papillary
- Septations, if present, that are thick (>2 cm)
- Color or power Doppler demonstration of flow in the solid component
- The presence of ascites (abnormal findings are any peritoneal fluid in postmenopausal women and more than a small amount of peritoneal fluid in premenopausal women)
- Peritoneal masses, enlarged nodes, or matted bowel (may be difficult to detect)

Treatment

The treatment of adnexal masses can be categorized as surgical (removal of the mass for pathologic diagnosis) or expectant management, which generally involves serial exams and ultrasounds to assure that the appearance of the mass does not become more concerning for malignancy. If a patient presents with an adnexal mass and an acute abdominal exam, such as the patient in the clinical encounter, your management will always be immediate surgical exploration. It is the asymptomatic adnexal masses whose management may vary depending on several factors. Here are some clinical guidelines to help with deciding between surgical and expectant management:

Premenopausal Therapy

Simple cysts smaller than 10 cm can be managed expectantly. Seventy percent will resolve spontaneously. Oral contraceptive pills may be prescribed to prevent ovulation and the formation of further cysts (6). All patients with an adnexal mass, especially if larger than 4 to 5 cm, should be given strong warnings about the symptoms of ovarian torsion and the importance of promptly treating this complication to avoid permanent adnexal damage. If the cyst is larger than 10 cm in size or exhibits any of the suspicious characteristics shown in the previous list, it should be surgically removed. Other findings that suggest malignancy and warrant surgical exploration include ascites, a CA-125 level >200 U/mL, suspicion for metastatic disease, or a first-degree relative with breast or ovarian cancer (6).

CLINICAL PEARL

An ovarian torsion is a surgical emergency. You should promptly intervene either by laparoscopy or laparotomy to avoid permanent adnexal damage. A torsed ovary can be reduced if there is no evidence of necrosis.

Postmenopausal Therapy

Postmenopausal women who are asymptomatic with a normal pelvic exam, a normal CA-125 finding, and a simple unilateral cyst <3 cm on ultrasound may be followed with serial ultrasounds and CA-125 examinations. Other size cutoffs that are commonly used are 4 and 5 cm. Postmenopausal women with a cyst >3 cm should have it surgically removed. This may be done laparoscopically in select patients.

Postmenopausal women with a symptomatic cyst, a CA-125 level >35 U/mL, ascites, a suspicion of metastatic disease, a history of a first-degree relative with breast or ovarian cancer, or a complex mass on ultrasound should undergo surgical intervention by a gynecologic oncologist (6).

EXTENDED IN-HOSPITAL MANAGEMENT

Patients with an adnexal mass that required emergent surgical intervention will need inpatient management postoperatively. Routine postoperative cares include the close monitoring of vital signs and urine output, pain control with intravenous pain medications until the patient is tolerating liquids, a slow advancement of diet as tolerated, and assistance with ambulation. A hematocrit level should be checked postoperatively to ensure that excessive blood loss during surgery did not occur.

DISPOSITION

Discharge Goals

Before a postoperative patient may be discharged home, she must meet certain criteria:

- The patient is afebrile with stable vital signs
- The patient maintains a stable hematocrit level
- The patient tolerates a regular diet
- The patient has a return of gastrointestinal function as demonstrated by the passing of flatus and/or bowel sounds
- The patient is ambulating
- The patient's pain is controlled on oral pain medications

Outpatient Care

If a patient has been operated on emergently to remove an adnexal mass, she will be seen in the clinic 4 weeks after discharge from the hospital for a postoperative check. This visit will include a discussion of how the patient has been feeling at home, an exam to ensure that the incision in healing, and a review of any pathology results from the surgery. If the surgical pathology is benign and her postoperative exam is normal, she can return to having annual exams. If there was malignancy found on pathology, the patient will require referral to a gynecologic oncologist.

- If a patient has an adnexal mass that is suspicious enough for malignancy to warrant surgical removal, outpatient care will include a preoperative visit and scheduling surgery.

If a patient has an adnexal mass that has been deemed safe for surveillance, she should be followed as an outpatient with serial exams and ultrasounds. The timing of this follow-up visit is variable, but one suggestion is at 3, 6, 9, and 12 months, and annually thereafter (6).

WHAT YOU NEED TO REMEMBER

- Adnexal masses are a common finding in women of all ages, and are a condition that all gynecologists should be comfortable diagnosing, managing, and treating.
- The causes of adnexal masses are numerous and differ among various age groups of women.
- An adnexal mass in postmenopausal women is considered to be cancerous until proven otherwise.
- Ultrasound is the best imaging modality for visualizing and characterizing an adnexal mass.
- CA-125 is neither sensitive nor specific as a screening test for ovarian cancer, but is useful as a marker to guide treatment.
- An adnexal mass can be treated with surgical removal or may be managed expectantly with serial exams and ultrasounds, depending on the acuity of the clinical presentation as well as the likelihood for malignancy.

REFERENCES

1. Hoffman MS. Differential diagnosis of the adnexal mass. http://www.uptodate. com. Accessed June 16, 2008.
2. Stenchever MA, Droegemueller W, Herbst AL, et al. *Comprehensive Gynecology.* 4th ed. St. Louis: Mosby; 2001:168–171, 955.
3. Growdon WB, Laufer MR. Ovarian and fallopian tube torsion. http://www. uptodate.com. Accessed June 16, 2008.
4. Cunningham FG, Leveno KJ, Bloom SL, et al. *Williams Obstetrics.* 22nd ed. New York: McGraw-Hill; 2005:124–125.

5. Norwitz ER, Schorge JO. *Obstetrics & Gynecology at a Glance*. Oxford: Blackwell; 2001:61.
6. Hoffman MS. Overview of the evaluation and management of adnexal masses. http://www.uptodate.com. Accessed June 16, 2008.

SUGGESTED READINGS

Oelsner G, Shashar D. Adnexal torsion. *Clin Obstet Gynecol*. 2006;49: 459–463.
Rock JA, Jones HW. *TeLinde's Operative Gynecology*. 9th ed. Philadelphia: Lippincott Williams & Wilkins; 2003:642–646.

Breast Disease

THE PATIENT ENCOUNTER

You are seeing a 42-year-old woman (G2P2002) in your office for evaluation of a breast lump that she discovered 2 weeks ago on breast self-exam. On examination, the mass is palpable at 10 o'clock in the left breast. The mass is mobile, well-circumscribed, and there is no nipple discharge, axillary lymphadenopathy, or clavicular lymphadenopathy.

OVERVIEW

Definition

Breast disease includes a wide variety of both benign disorders and malignant conditions. The ranges of symptoms for which women may consult their physician include breast masses, breast pain or mastalgia, nipple discharge, and mastitis. This chapter will review common benign breast disorders, malignant breast disease, and strategies for the management of these conditions.

Pathophysiology

Breast tissue undergoes many changes throughout a woman's lifetime. Both stromal cells and epithelial cells are influenced by a variety of hormones and growth factors. During puberty, rising estradiol and progesterone levels initiate breast development, and a treelike network of ducts and glands develops. In the fully mature breast, cyclic changes occur each month during the menstrual cycle. During the luteal phase, the breast may increase in size by up to 15% because of cell proliferation. After menopause, when estrogen and progesterone levels are low, the number of lobules present in a woman's breast tissue begins to decrease (1).

Epidemiology

Approximately one fourth of women will be affected by breast disease at some point during their lifetime (1). Mastalgia, or breast pain, has been reported by as many as 60% of women, and as many as 80% of premenopausal women may experience nipple discharge with significant breast manipulation (1). In the United States, the overall lifetime risk for developing breast cancer is one in eight; it is the second leading cause of cancer death among women (2).

Etiology

It is helpful to divide the etiology of breast disease into categories by symptoms.

Mastalgia

Breast pain may either manifest as cyclic or noncyclic pain. The most common cause of severe cyclic breast pain is fibrocystic change. This condition is characterized by diffuse "lumpy-bumpy" changes in the breast on examination and pain that occurs during the luteal phase of the menstrual cycle. Many women experience mild pain during the luteal phase, but only 11% experience moderate-to-severe pain (1). It is controversial whether factors such as caffeine, iodine deficiency, and the percentage of diet from fat play a role in fibrocystic change (1).

Another cause of breast pain is mastitis. This is a condition common during the first 3 months postpartum in breast-feeding women. Patients typically present with fever, myalgias, local inflammation, erythema, and pain. Mastitis is commonly caused by skin flora that causes cellulitis in the connective tissue of the mammary glands. Cracks or fissures in the nipple due to improper nursing techniques combined with stress and fatigue predispose postpartum women to this condition (3). For many women, physical factors contribute to noncyclic breast pain. Physical causes of breast pain include pain from a poorly fitting bra, the stretching of Cooper's ligaments in women with pendulous breasts, or fat necrosis from trauma. A rare condition known as Mondor disease also causes breast pain. Women with Mondor disease usually present with a tender, cordlike structure in the breast, which is caused by a blood clot in one of the superficial veins in the breast. When a patient complains of breast pain, the physician must carefully evaluate the patient for conditions that might cause pain that are unrelated to the breast, such as coronary artery disease, costochondritis, hiatal hernias, and cholelithiasis.

Nipple Discharge

Nipple discharge may be galactorrhea that is caused by hyperprolactinemia. Hyperprolactinemia may be caused by a pituitary tumor, hypothyroidism, or medications, including oral contraceptives and certain psychiatric medications. Other causes of nipple discharge are intraductal papillomas, fibrocystic changes, ductal ectasia, Paget disease of the breast, and breast cancer. Intraductal papillomas are benign tumors of the epithelium of the mammary glands. They are typically small lesions that are very difficult to palpate and located under the areola. Mammary ductal ectasia is a condition of middle-aged women who may present with discharge and a palpable mass. They also might have nipple inversion or retraction. It may be noticed on a mammogram in an asymptomatic woman because microcalcifications may be seen. Paget disease of the breast presents with nipple lesions that appear to be similar to eczema.

These skin changes are associated with an underlying breast malignancy, ranging from ductal carcinoma in situ to metastatic ductal carcinoma.

Although nipple discharge most commonly is a symptom of a benign condition, nipple discharge is suspected to be pathologic if it is persistent, contains blood, or arises from a single duct. Patient age also plays an important role in predicting the cause of nipple discharge, and the provider's suspicion for malignancy should increase when an older woman presents with nipple discharge as a symptom. Nipple discharge is present in fewer than 3% of patients with breast carcinoma and 10% to 15% of women with benign breast disease (4).

Breast Mass

For women who present with a solitary breast mass, the most common etiology depends on the patients' age. In women younger than age 30, the most common cause of a breast mass is a benign fibroadenoma. In women between the ages of 30 and 50, causes include fibroadenomas, cysts, ductal hyperplasia, both usual and atypical, and atypical lobular hyperplasia. In women older than age 50, the most common lesions include cysts, ductal carcinoma in situ, and invasive breast cancer.

ACUTE MANAGEMENT AND WORKUP

It is important to realize that women who present to their physician for the evaluation of a complaint related to their breasts are often frightened that they might have breast cancer, and as a result are often very anxious about their condition.

The First 15 Minutes

If you suspect a benign condition, it is important to assess the situation accurately to reassure the patient, and to help the patient develop realistic expectations about her condition if you suspect she might have breast cancer.

Initial Assessment

A multidisciplinary approach is necessary to properly evaluate, treat, and manage breast complaints. The primary physician evaluating the mass will ultimately maintain continuity of care throughout the process and should be well versed in the most commonly used diagnostic algorithms to ensure that steps do not get missed as the patient goes from one provider to another.

Admission Criteria and Level of Care Criteria

Unless the source of disease is infectious in nature, most breast pathology is managed in an outpatient setting. Patients with severe postpartum mastitis and/or the presence of an abscess may require hospitalization for treatment with intravenous antibiotics and surgical drainage of the abscess.

The First Few Hours

A detailed description of your initial clinical findings will help track the progress of disease. A thorough history and physical exam can identify risk factors that will further stratify the patient's prognosis.

History

You should always begin with a thorough patient history and breast exam. The symptoms the patient is experiencing should be characterized and risk factors for breast cancer should be identified. You should obtain the patient's age at the following markers: menarche, the first live birth, and menopause. The presence of a family history of breast cancer or ovarian cancer and the family member's age at diagnosis should be determined. If the patient has had any previous breast biopsies, you need to review the results. Finally, you should determine if the patient has used hormone replacement therapy in the past.

Physical Examination

The breast exam should consist of the following steps:

1. Palpation of all four quadrants of the breast with the patient sitting and supine
2. Identification of lymphadenopathy
3. Examination of the skin, axilla and areola, and determination of the degree of symmetry in both breasts
4. Examination of the nipple for any discharge. Determination of whether discharge is from one or multiple ducts, and if it is watery, bloody, clear, blue-black, green, or milky
5. Examination for chest wall pain

When a mass is found on the physical exam, there are certain characteristics that are more commonly found in masses that are malignant. If a mass is hard, is fixed to the chest wall, has an irregular border, is larger than 2 cm in size, or presents with overlying changes in the skin, such as dimpling, the lesion is more likely to be malignant than if the mass is soft, small, and mobile with regular borders.

Labs and Tests to Consider

The next step in management depends on the presenting complaint and the age of the patient. For women under the age of 35 with a discrete breast mass that is not suspicious for malignancy, ultrasonography is the next step in the evaluation. For women older than age 35 or if the mass is suspicious for malignancy, a mammogram is the appropriate diagnostic test.

Treatment

The next step depends on the imaging findings, as shown in Figure 20-1. If a lesion is found to be cystic on ultrasound, the fluid may be aspirated. For

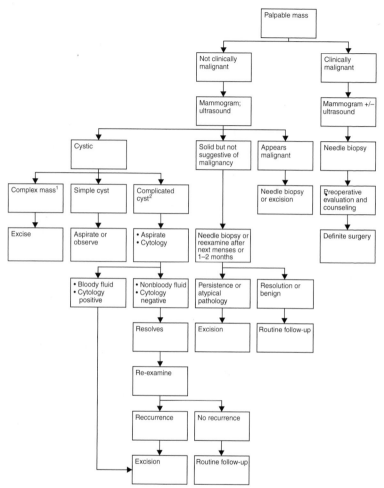

FIGURE 20-1: Management of patients with a breast mass.

women found to have a solid mass, generally either a fine-needle aspiration or a core needle biopsy is performed for cytologic or histologic diagnosis of the lesion.

Fibroadenomas may be treated by excision. Thirty percent of fibroadenomas will disappear and 10% to 12% become smaller if they are followed for many years, so they do not require removal in all women. Fibroadenomas also recur in 20% of women in whom they are removed (4). Most women prefer to have the fibroadenoma excised rather than followed conservatively.

The treatment of intraductal papillomas usually involves resection of the involved duct and a small amount of surrounding tissue.

Acute postpartum mastitis is generally managed with a course of oral antibiotics that cover gram-positive microbes, specifically dicloxacillin. For women with a penicillin allergy, azithromycin may be an alternative regimen. The woman should be encouraged to continue breast-feeding. A patient should be evaluated for a breast abscess if she fails to respond to oral antibiotics, has recurrent mastitis, or has a clinically suspicious lesion.

If a patient is found to have galactorrhea due to thyroid dysfunction, this condition should be treated. If the prolactin level is elevated because of a pituitary adenoma, she should be treated for this condition. If the patient's thyroid and prolactin levels are normal, and medications are ruled out as a cause, the patient may be treated with a dopamine agonist, such as bromocriptine or cabergoline for symptomatic relief. For women who have bloody nipple discharge and there is a clinically suspicious mass, the next step in your evaluation may include galactography, or imaging of the ducts of the breast using dye that will identify any lesions located within the ducts. Any lesions identified on galactography should be removed because of the risk of invasive cancer.

Patients who are diagnosed with invasive breast cancer or carcinoma in situ should undergo appropriate evaluation with a surgeon who treats women with breast cancer to make a decision regarding the appropriate type of treatment. Breast cancer is typically treated surgically, although the correct surgery for each patient remains a decision among the provider, the patient, and the patient's family.

EXTENDED IN-HOSPITAL MANAGEMENT

The appropriate management of breast disease depends on the patient's diagnosis. The majority of women with benign breast disease will not require hospitalization and can be managed as outpatients. Women who are diagnosed with breast cancer will often require hospitalization for recovery from surgical procedures such as mastectomies and breast-reconstructive surgery.

DISPOSITION
Discharge Goals

Infectious processes are treated with intravenous antibiotics until the patient has been afebrile for at least 48 hours. In the case of a breast mass lumpectomy, the patient should be treated on an outpatient basis. Those patients are sent home with a longer course of continued antibiotics. Major surgical procedures (such as a mastectomy) will be performed by a surgical oncologist.

Outpatient Care

For women with fibrocystic change, management strategies include wearing a support bra both day and night. For some women, diuretics administered during the premenstrual period or the administration of oral contraceptives may provide relief. There is only one medication that is approved for the treatment of cyclic mastalgia, danazol, which is a gonadotropin-releasing hormone antagonist. Danazol relieves symptoms and decreases breast masses in 90% of patients, and side effects, such as menopausal symptoms and bone loss, can be severe (4). Tamoxifen has also been used to treat mastalgia. Finally, alternative remedies such as evening primrose oil have been studied for the treatment of mastalgia, with conflicting results (1).

Breast Cancer Screening

Breast cancer screening techniques include breast self-exam, clinical breast exam, mammography, and breast magnetic resonance imaging. Although the evidence for breast self-exam is limited, it has the benefit of detecting additional breast cancers and should be recommended (5).

CLINICAL PEARL

A yearly clinical breast exam should be performed as part of the routine physical exam. Routine screening with mammography is recommended every 1 to 2 years for women between the ages of 40 and 49 and yearly thereafter (5).

Recently, breast magnetic resonance imaging has been demonstrated to be an effective screening technique in certain high-risk women.

WHAT YOU NEED TO REMEMBER

- In the United States, the lifetime risk of breast cancer for women is one in eight.
- The most common cause of bloody nipple discharge is an intraductal papilloma.
- The most common cause of a breast mass in young women is a benign fibroadenoma.
- The most common cause of cyclic breast pain is fibrocystic change.

- In a woman with a breast mass, the evaluation should include a combination of breast exam, ultrasound, and mammography.
- Postpartum women with mastitis should continue to breast-feed.
- Women should be taught breast self-exam techniques and should have yearly clinical breast exams.
- Women should start having mammograms every 1 to 2 years at the age of 40 and yearly at the age of 50 for breast cancer screening.

REFERENCES

1. Santen RJ, Mansel R. Benign breast disorders. *N Engl J Med.* 2005;353:275–285.
2. Berek JS, Hacker NF. *Practical Gynecologic Oncology.* 4th ed. Philadelphia: Lippincott Williams & Wilkins; 2005:626–662.
3. Guray M, Sahin A. Benign breast diseases: classification, diagnosis and management. *Oncologist.* 2006;11:435–449.
4. Katz VL, Lentz GM, Lobo RA, et al. *Comprehensive Gynecology.* 5th ed. Philadelphia: Mosby Elsevier; 2007:330–334.
5. American College of Obstetricians and Gynecologists. ACOG practice bulletin number 42: screening for breast cancer, April 2003. *Obstet Gynecol.* 2003;101: 821–832.

Endometriosis

THE PATIENT ENCOUNTER

You are called to the emergency department to see one of your patients who has presented there complaining of pelvic pain. The patient is a 32-year-old woman (G0P0) who you saw in the office for the first time 2 weeks ago. She had reported worsening pelvic pain for the past 7 years. She stated that it began with dysmenorrhea, which then progressed to pain outside of menses; now she has significant dyspareunia and painful bowel movements as well. Upon examination that day, you noted a 5-cm, right-sided adnexal mass, and some tenderness and nodularity along her uterosacral ligaments.

OVERVIEW

Definition

Endometriosis is a chronic condition that is characterized by the growth of endometrial glands and stroma in sites other than the uterus. It may cause pelvic pain and/or infertility, although it may also be asymptomatic. Endometriosis may be noted on peritoneal surfaces throughout the abdomen and pelvis, in the ovaries, and in surgical scars, and it may involve the bladder or bowel; it has even been documented in distant sites such as the thorax.

Pathophysiology

The extrauterine glands and stroma in the patient with endometriosis are estrogen-dependent; thus, endometriosis is generally not found in premenarchal girls. These implants are often functional, causing pain at the time of the patient's menses. Over time, inflammation and scarring may ensue, which can distort pelvic anatomy, potentially causing pain and infertility. As the inflammation and scarring progress, the patient's pain may be noted at any time during her menstrual cycle, not confined to menses. Lesions may be present on the surface of the peritoneum and of organs, or they may infiltrate deeply. It has been noted, however, that often the extent of disease is not related to the extent of pain, although it has some relation to infertility. Grossly, lesions of endometriosis can have variable appearances. Classically, the term *powder-burn lesion* has been used to describe black or dark brown puckered lesions noted on the peritoneum, the serosa, or the ovaries.

Endometriotic lesions can also be clear, red, blue-black, yellow, brown, or white. Ovarian endometriosis may appear on the surface of the ovary, but also may present as an endometrioma, a cyst filled with blood, fluid, and menstrual debris, often termed a *chocolate cyst*. The American Society for Reproductive Medicine has developed a classification system for endometriosis, which underwent its third revision in 1996 (Table 21-1). The classification is useful in providing a standardized method of communicating operative findings; however, it correlates poorly with the pain symptoms.

Histologic examination remains the gold standard for the diagnosis of endometriosis, especially of lesions that do not have a classic appearance.

TABLE 21-1
American Society for Reproductive Medicine Classification System for Endometriosis

Patient's name _____ Date _____

Stage I (minimal) — 1–5
Stage II (mild) — 6–15
Stage III (moderate) — 16–40
Stage IV (severe) — >40
Total _____

Laparoscopy____ Laparotomy _____ Photography_____
Recommended treatment _____
_____
Prognosis _____

	Endometriosis	<1 cm	1–3 cm	>3 cm
Peritoneum	Superficial	1	2	4
	Deep	2	4	5
Ovary	R Superficial	1	2	4
	Deep	4	16	20
	L Superficial	1	2	4
	Deep	4	15	20
	Posterior cul-de-sac obliteration	Partial		Complete
		4		40
	Adhesions	<1/3 Enclosure	1/3–2/3 Enclosure	>2/3 Enclosure
Ovary	R Filmy	1	2	4
	Dense	4	8	16
	L Filmy	1	2	4
	Dense	4	8	15
Tube	R Filmy	1	2	4
	Dense	4*	8*	16
	L Filmy	1	2	4
	Dense	4*	5*	16

* If the fimbriated end of the fallopian tube is completely enclosed, change the point assignment to 15. Denote appearance of superficial implant types as red [(R), red, red-pink, flamelike, vesicular blobs, clear vesicles], white [(W), opacifications, peritoneal defects, yellow-brown, or black [(B), black, hemosiderin deposits, blue]. Denote percent of total described as R__%, W__%, and B__%. Total should equal 100%.

The specimen must have two of the following criteria for the pathologist to diagnose endometriosis:

- Endometrial epithelium
- Endometrial glands
- Endometrial stroma
- Hemosiderin-laden macrophages

In addition, endometriosis has been identified as an independent risk factor for epithelial ovarian cancer, conferring a modest increase in risk, with the risk of malignant transformation of ovarian endometriosis estimated at 2.5%.

Epidemiology

The prevalence of endometriosis in the general population is not known but is estimated to range between 6% and 10%. For subsets of women who are at higher risk for endometriosis, the incidence is better appreciated. In women with chronic pelvic pain, endometriosis is diagnosed in approximately one third of women who undergo surgical evaluation. Infertile women have endometriosis found at laparoscopy in approximately 30% to 50% of cases (1). It is most commonly diagnosed between the ages of 25 and 35 years. A familial association of endometriosis has been documented, with a 7% risk of developing disease in first-degree relatives. The proposed inheritance is multifactorial, likely involving the interplay of several genes with each other and with environmental factors.

Etiology

The pathogenesis of endometriosis remains unclear. Leading theories have traditionally included the following: retrograde menstruation, hematogenous or lymphatogenous transport, and coelomic metaplasia. The theory of retrograde menstruation postulates that endometriosis may arise from the direct implantation of menstrual debris that flows through the fallopian tubes and into the peritoneal cavity. It has been well documented that women with outflow obstruction that occurs congenitally, such as imperforate hymen or cervical atresia, are more likely to develop endometriosis. However, it has also been noted that the incidence of retrograde menstruation is the same in women with and without endometriosis, suggesting that something else must play a role. There is some evidence that altered immune surveillance may play a role in the pathogenesis of the disease. The theory of hematogenous or lymphatogenous spread has been used to explain those cases in which endometriosis occurs in distant sites, such as the thorax. Coelomic metaplasia refers to the theory that peritoneal cells may be able to differentiate into the endometrium. Additionally, there is a theory that endometrial cells may be directly transplanted into cesarean section scars, episiotomy sites, and other surgical sites.

ACUTE MANAGEMENT AND WORKUP

Endometriosis is typically managed as a chronic condition; however, acute issues may be encountered. An ovarian endometrioma can cause acute pain from the size and pressure of the mass or it may cause acute pain from torsion or rupture of the mass. The classic history in these scenarios is one of sudden onset of severe pelvic pain. A ruptured cyst can cause severe pain and may also cause a hemoperitoneum; the bleeding may resolve on its own, but sometimes it can be life-threatening and will necessitate surgical intervention. It should be noted, however, that endometriomas are generally thick-walled and often adhere to the pelvic side wall or the back of the uterus; thus, it is uncommon that they rupture or undergo torsion, although it does happen.

The First 15 Minutes

The goals of management of the patient who presents with acute pelvic pain are the same whether or not the patient has endometriosis. The patient's hemodynamic stability is first assessed, life-threatening diagnoses are ruled out, and then a careful evaluation is performed to obtain the diagnosis and decide on a course of management. The differential diagnosis for acute pelvic pain is quite broad and may involve any pelvic organ including the bowel, bladder, ureters, uterus, tubes, and ovaries. The most common emergent diagnoses are ectopic pregnancy, ovarian torsion, ruptured ovarian cyst, pelvic inflammatory disease, and appendicitis. Your patient with endometriosis who presents with acute pelvic pain to the emergency department is most often going to be in the reproductive age group; therefore, the preservation of fertility should be kept in mind.

Initial Assessment

Your initial assessment involves the following steps:

- First, observe the patient. Does she appear ill? Is she writhing in pain? Is she pale and diaphoretic? Check the patient's vital signs and make sure the patient is not hypotensive or tachycardic.
- Make sure the patient is not pregnant by obtaining a urine pregnancy test to rule out the possibility of ectopic pregnancy.
- Take a focused history. Ask about the onset, location, quality, and duration of the pain and any exacerbating or alleviating factors. Ask about any associated symptoms such as nausea, vomiting, fever, or gastrointestinal or urinary symptoms.
- Examine the abdomen. Look, listen, percuss, and palpate. Does the patient appear distended? Does she have hypoactive bowel sounds? Is the abdomen tympanitic? Is it rigid, with peritoneal signs such as involuntary guarding and rebound?

Admission Criteria and Level of Care Criteria

The next step in the care of the patient seen on an emergent basis is to triage her based on your initial assessment of her condition. Keep in mind that the condition of the patient may change as she is observed.

Option 1: Stable Condition

The patient has minimal-to-mild pain on examination. The abdominal and pelvic exams reveal no obvious abnormalities. The vital signs are normal and the patient has a negative pregnancy test. The workup can proceed to determine diagnosis; this will likely include pelvic ultrasound and may be performed as an outpatient with close follow-up.

Option 2: Fair Condition

The patient has moderate pain on examination, but no peritoneal signs. The vital signs are stable. The workup must continue until the most likely diagnosis is established and a plan of care may then be determined.

Option 3: Critical Condition

The patient has peritoneal signs on examination. Vital signs demonstrate hypotension or tachycardia. This patient has a surgical abdomen; if she has a positive pregnancy test, the likely diagnosis is ectopic pregnancy, although a ruptured cyst may also be present. If the patient is febrile with peritonitis on examination, the likely diagnosis is either a perforated appendix or fulminant pelvic inflammatory disease. Two large-bore intravenous lines should be available, with a bolus of saline or lactated Ringer solution administered. You should prepare your patient for surgery. If the patient's condition permits, you can perform a quick bedside ultrasound to assess for free fluid.

The First Few Hours

After triaging the patient according to her condition, the next step is to continue with evaluation and management. At this point, the patient with a benign exam will likely be discharged home with outpatient appointments for ultrasound and follow-up. The patient in critical condition with an acute abdomen will have proceeded to surgery. Most patients, however, will fall into the middle category and will require further assessment.

History

At this point, an initial brief history has already been obtained so the symptoms should be further delineated. You should carefully question your patient about the chronicity of pain and its association with menses, intercourse, bowel movements, and urination. A sexual history should be obtained; a history of sexually transmitted diseases should be ascertained, as should the circumstances surrounding those diagnoses. Many women with endometriosis have been diagnosed with pelvic inflammatory disease multiple times in their past, so documentation of positive cervical cultures or of laparoscopy findings is important.

Physical Examination

The pelvic exam should be performed with attention to the presence of cervical motion tenderness, adnexal masses or tenderness, uterine position, and contour. The rectovaginal septum and uterosacral ligaments should be assessed for nodularity, which is often present in more advanced cases of endometriosis.

Labs and Tests to Consider

Patients presenting with acute pelvic pain should first undergo pregnancy testing to rule out ectopic gestation. Other tests that are often helpful include the following:

- Complete blood count (to evaluate hemoglobin and white blood cell count)
- Gonococcal and chlamydial cultures (to evaluate for pelvic inflammatory disease)
- Urinalysis (to evaluate for urinary tract infection or renal colic)
- Hemoccult (to evaluate for diverticular disease or other gastrointestinal disease)
- Serum CA-125 (if an adnexal mass is present, this test is not helpful emergently but may be of use for long-term management)

Imaging

Key imaging tests include pelvic ultrasound and computed tomography scan. Pelvic ultrasound is useful in assessing for ectopic pregnancy, adnexal masses, ovarian torsion, and evidence of pelvic inflammatory disease. A computed tomography scan is more sensitive and specific than ultrasound for evaluation of the appendix.

Treatment

Options for therapy include expectant, medical (Table 21-2), or surgical management, or a combination of medical and surgical management. The patient who desires fertility in the near future should not be managed medically.

Medical Management

The asymptomatic patient who is noted to have endometriosis as an incidental finding may reasonably be managed expectantly, particularly in those women who have completed childbearing. The difficulty lies in counseling a woman with asymptomatic endometriosis who desires future fertility. The evidence supporting medical therapy to prevent progression of disease and

TABLE 21-2

Medical Treatment Options for Endometriosis

Drug	Mechanism of Action	Length of Treatment Recommended	Adverse Events	Notes
Medroxyprogesterone acetate/progestagens	Ovarian suppression	Long term	Weight gain, bloating, acne, irregular bleeding	May be given orally or by intramuscular or subcutaneous depot injection
Danazol	Ovarian suppression	6–9 months	Weight gain, bloating, acne, hirsutism, skin rashes	Adverse effects on lipid profiles
Oral contraceptive	Ovarian suppression	Long term	Nausea, headaches	Can be used to avoid menstruation by skipping placebo pills

| GnRH analogue | Ovarian suppression by competitive inhibitor of GnRH analogue | 6 months | Hot flushes, other symptoms of hypoestrogenism | By injection or nasal spray only |
| Levonorgestrel intrauterine system | Endometrial suppression, ovarian suppression in some women | Long term use, but change every 5 years | Irregular bleeding | Also reduces menstrual blood loss |

GnRH, gonadotropin-releasing hormone.

to thereby improve fertility is lacking; however, many studies do report a reduced incidence of endometriosis in women who use oral contraceptives.

A patient with moderate-to-severe pain can undergo a trial of oral contraceptives but may require a gonadotropin-releasing hormone (GnRH) agonist, which will induce a menopausal state temporarily. These can be given as an intranasal spray or more commonly as intramuscular injections every 1 to 3 months.

CLINICAL PEARL

A GnRH agonist will temporarily induce a menopausal state. The side effects are mitigated by giving add-back therapy of progestin or estrogen/progestin. A course of therapy will typically last no longer than 6 months.

Progestational agents may also be used in a patient with significant pain. These are formulated as depot medroxyprogesterone acetate, are given intramuscularly or subcutaneously, or are given as high-dose oral agents. They induce a pseudopregnancy state and side effects include weight gain, irregular bleeding, and mood changes. The levonorgestrel intrauterine contraceptive has also been used to improve pain and provide contraception for women with endometriosis with fewer side effects.

Danazol, which is an androgen, has also been found effective in treating pain and reducing the size of implants. The associated side effects include hirsutism, weight gain, acne, oily skin, deepening of the voice, and elevated liver enzymes. The side effects can only be moderated by decreasing the dose, so patients are often instead treated with a GnRH agonist with add-back therapy.

Surgical Management

Surgical therapy is indicated when the patient's symptoms are severe and incapacitating, or are acute, such as is found in rupture or torsion of an endometrioma. Surgery is also appropriate when the patient's symptoms have not responded to medical therapy or the patient declines hormonal management.

Surgical management can be conservative, preserving the uterus and ovaries, or it can be definitive, removing the uterus with or without removal of the ovaries. Conservative treatment includes destroying visible endometriotic implants and restoring normal anatomy by lysing adhesions and removing endometriomas. Conservative surgical therapy is often followed by medical management to try to prolong the pain-free interval if the patient does not desire immediate fertility. Definitive therapy can be employed when the patient has completed childbearing. Removal of the ovaries is largely dependent on the patient's age, but ovaries that are severely damaged by endometriosis may require removal at a young age, and these patients may require hormonal therapy postoperatively.

EXTENDED IN-HOSPITAL MANAGEMENT

As stated previously, endometriosis is typically managed as a chronic condition, although there are some patients with extensive disease who remain asymptomatic. It is also important to remember that although it is suggested that endometriosis is progressive for most women, this may not always be the case.

DISPOSITION

Discharge Goals

If surgical management is initiated, a standard postoperative treatment plan should be initiated. Pain control and counseling about future fertility should be addressed prior to discharge.

Outpatient Care

A patient with mild pelvic pain may be managed either with analgesics or with oral contraceptives, if there is no contraindication present for oral contraceptive use. Nonsteroidal anti-inflammatory drugs have been documented to be effective in the treatment of primary dysmenorrhea, but are not likely to be effective in a patient with endometriosis who has greater than minimal pain. The oral contraceptives cause decidualization and atrophy of the endometrium, including the ectopic endometrium, and have the additional benefits of providing contraception, and may be used in the long term.

Patients with endometriosis should have serial evaluations every 4 to 6 months to assess pain control and symptomatology. The most difficult aspect of treating patients with chronic pain is the tendency of patients to be bounced around from one provider to another.

WHAT YOU NEED TO REMEMBER

- Endometriosis is a chronic condition associated with pelvic pain and infertility, and is characterized by the presence of endometrial tissue outside the uterine cavity.
- Laparoscopy with biopsy has long been considered the gold standard for diagnosis.

- Management can be medical or surgical, or a combination of both.
- Medical therapy should be avoided in women actively trying to conceive.
- The combined oral contraceptive pill is often the first-line therapy.
- Medical therapies include oral contraceptives, progestational agents such as depot medroxyprogesterone acetate, GnRH agonists, and Danazol. All have been shown to improve pain symptoms.
- Surgical management can be conservative, preserving the uterus and ovaries, or definitive.

REFERENCE

1. Katz VL, Lentz GM, Lobo RA, et al. *Comprehensive Gynecology.* 5th ed. Philadelphia: Mosby Elsevier; 2007.

SUGGESTED READINGS

American College of Obstetricians and Gynecologists. ACOG committee opinion number 310: endometriosis in adolescents. *Obstet Gynecol.* 2005;105:921–927.

Farquhar C. Endometriosis. *Br Med J.* 2007;334;249–253.

Giudice LC, Kao LC. Endometriosis. *Lancet.* 2004;364;1789–1799.

Lobo RA. Endometriosis. In: Katz VL, Lentz GM, Lobo RA, Gershenson DM, eds. *Comprehensive Gynecology.* 5th ed. Philadelphia: Mosby; 2007:473–501.

Moghissi KS, Winkel CA. Medical management of endometriosis (practice bulletin number 11). ACOG Compendium of Selected Publications 2008:1036–1048. Available at: www.acog.org/publications/educational_bulletins/pb011.cfm. Accessed July 21, 2008.

Amenorrhea

THE PATIENT ENCOUNTER

Your next patient is a 17-year-old adolescent girl (G0P0) who presents stating that she has never had a period. You are seeing her for the first time as a referral from her primary care provider. She reports that she is sexually active and is healthy with no medical problems.

OVERVIEW

Definitions

Primary amenorrhea is characterized by a complete absence of menses by age 14 and no development of secondary sexual characteristics (breasts or pubic hair). It is also characterized by a lack of period by age 16 and the presence of secondary sexual characteristics.

Women with secondary amenorrhea have no menses for 6 months after having had previous menstrual cycles. This condition also includes women with previous menstrual cycles who have not had a menses for three cycles.

This chapter will discuss the etiology and workup for patients presenting with amenorrhea.

Pathophysiology

When evaluating a patient with amenorrhea, *the first step is to rule out pregnancy*. The remaining causes of amenorrhea are primarily due to dysfunction of the hypothalamic pituitary axis (i.e., gonadotropin-releasing hormone, follicle-stimulating hormone [FSH], and luteinizing hormone), ovarian dysfunction, an outflow tract abnormality or other endocrinopathies (i.e., hypothyroidism, hyperprolactinemia).

CLINICAL PEARL

Always be sure to rule out pregnancy in anyone of reproductive age complaining of amenorrhea.

Epidemiology

Although nearly 5% of all menstruating women will experience some period of secondary amenorrhea over the course of their reproductive lives, prolonged secondary amenorrhea (>6 months) occurs in only 0.7% of reproductive-age women (1). In the case of secondary amenorrhea, a majority of these findings have been linked to a hypothalamic disorder.

Etiology

The etiology of amenorrhea can be divided into three broad categories: hypergonadotropic hypogonadism, hypogonadotropic hypogonadism, and eugonadism. Patients with hypergonadotropic hypogonadism have an elevated FSH level, which demonstrates normal pituitary function and ovarian dysfunction. This group accounts for 50% of cases of amenorrhea. Patients with hypogonadotropic hypogonadism have a decreased FSH level, likely caused by a disruption in the hypothalamic pituitary axis. Patients with eugonadism have normal FSH and estrogen levels and generally have anatomic or endocrine abnormalities. Table 22-1 provides a list of etiologies of amenorrhea.

ACUTE MANAGEMENT AND WORKUP

Amenorrhea is rarely an acute event. Menstrual irregularity is frustrating but a systematic evaluation will usually yield a diagnosis.

The First 15 Minutes

The most important condition to exclude in the first 15 minutes is pregnancy-induced amenorrhea.

Initial Assessment

A simple urine pregnancy test is sufficient for diagnosing pregnancy. The initial 15 minutes will also give you a sense of how bothered the patient is about her loss of menses.

The First Few Hours

A systematic evaluation with a thorough physical exam will narrow the extensive differential diagnosis and aid in establishing the proper diagnosis.

History

When evaluating a patient for amenorrhea, you should always obtain a thorough history. Make sure to ascertain the following information:

- Has the patient ever had a menstrual period? (Distinguish between primary versus secondary amenorrhea.)

TABLE 22-1

Causes of Amenorrhea

Hypergonadotropic Hypogonadism	Hypogonadotropic Hypogonadism	Eugonadism
• Gonadal dysgenesis	• Constitutional delay	• Chronic anovulation (PCOS, CAH)
• Turner syndrome (45 X)	• Anorexia, weight loss	• Cushing syndrome
• Swyer syndrome (46 XY)	• Extreme exercise	• Imperforate hymen
• Premature ovarian failure	• CNS neoplasm	• Transverse vaginal septum
• History of radiation/chemo	• Kallmann syndrome	• Mullerian agenesis
	• Sheehan syndrome	• Androgen resistance
	• Idiopathic	• Asherman syndrome

PCOS, polycystic ovary syndrome; CAH, congenital adrenal hyperplasia.

- Is the patient sexually active? (The answer helps rule out whether or not the patient is pregnant.)
- What is the patient's social situation? (Include questions about diet, exercise, and stress.)
- Has the patient experienced any neurologic changes (i.e., CNS abnormalities)?
- Has the patient experienced any exposure to medications or radiation or chemotherapy?
- Does the patient have a history of previous pregnancies or surgeries? (Include questions about Sheehan syndrome and Asherman syndrome.)

Physical Examination

The next step in the patient evaluation is the physical exam. Evaluate the following:

- Note the patient's height, weight, and general appearance.
- Does the patient have breast development? (The presence of breasts demonstrates the patient's estrogen status.)
- What is the distribution of hair growth? Are there signs of hirsutism?
- Is there a presence or an absence of a uterus, vagina, imperforate hymen, and vaginal septum?

Labs and Tests to Consider

Once a history is obtained and you complete the physical exam, the following initial tests will help guide the remainder of the patient's workup: beta-human chorionic gonadotropin (β-hCG), thyrotropin (TSH), prolactin, FSH, and a progesterone challenge test. Pregnancy is the most common cause of amenorrhea. Assuming that the TSH and prolactin levels are normal and the β-hCG is negative, the remainder of the workup will be directed based on the patient's history and physical exam findings, FSH, and progesterone challenge test. The progesterone challenge test is an administration of progesterone to the patient for 5 days. After stopping the administration of progesterone, if the patient has a withdrawal bleed, her ovaries are producing estrogen. If not, she is either not producing enough estrogen for endometrial proliferation or she could have an anatomic outflow tract abnormality (Fig. 22-1).

Treatment

The presence or absence of breasts and a uterus will help you categorize the appropriate diagnoses and facilitate the respective treatment plans.

Breasts Absent and Uterus Present

In these patients, the FSH level will determine whether the lack of ovarian production is a result of hypothalamic pituitary dysfunction or a gonadal

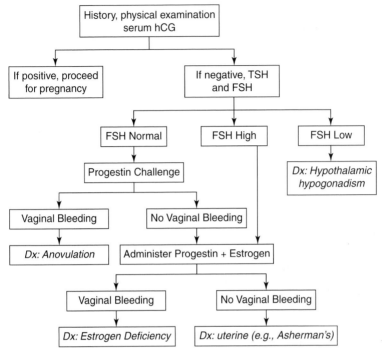

FIGURE 22-1: Approach to evaluating secondary amenorrhea.

disorder. An elevated FSH level reveals hypergonadotropic hypogonadism (Table 22-1); a karyotype should be ordered to determine the cause of gonadal dysfunction. If the karyotype is 45 X,O, then the diagnosis is Turner syndrome. Patients with this condition have fibrous gonadal streaks without follicles at birth. These patients can also have characteristic physical findings of short stature, webbing of the neck, and coarctation of the aorta. Most of these patients will require exogenous estrogen replacement. Patients with a 46 X,Y karyotype have Swyer syndrome. They are phenotypic females with a normal müllerian system and gonadal streaks. The cause of Swyer syndrome is the lack of a normal functioning sex region on the Y chromosome. Because there is a 30% risk of developing gonadoblastoma and dysgerminoma, these patients should undergo a gonadectomy. Patients with a normal karyotype likely have either premature ovarian failure or a history of radiation or chemotherapy, which can be differentiated based on their history.

In patients with a low FSH level, which represents hypogonadotropic hypogonadism, the patient's history will help to differentiate the cause.

The most common cause is a constitutional delay of puberty. If the patient history and physical exam are consistent with anorexia, severe weight loss, or extreme exercising, her diagnosis can be made, but magnetic resonance imaging should be considered to rule out CNS lesions. Kallmann syndrome is another cause of hypogonadotropic hypogonadism due to a defect in the *KALL* gene that leads to a disruption in the migration of gonadotropin-releasing hormone neurons. These patients can also have anosmia and midline facial defects. If the patient has a history of a postpartum hemorrhage, a diagnosis of Sheehan syndrome should be considered.

Breasts Present and Uterus Absent

The two causes for eugonadal patients with the absence of a uterus are androgen resistance and congenital absence of the uterus. Obtaining karyotype and testosterone levels should be ordered for these patients. Patients with a karyotype of 46 X,Y and male levels of testosterone have androgen resistance. On physical exam, they should have a blind vaginal pouch and a lack of pubic hair. Patients with a normal 46 X,X karyotype and female levels of testosterone have müllerian agenesis. These patients may also have cardiac, renal, or skeletal abnormalities that should warrant further evaluation.

Breasts Present and Uterus Present

For patients with primary amenorrhea who have the presence of a uterus and breasts, they likely have an anatomic outflow tract abnormality. The difference between an imperforate hymen and a transverse vaginal septum should be distinguished by physical exam. Both can be treated surgically. Other causes for patients with both breasts and uterus present are likely to be secondary amenorrhea. Patients with Asherman syndrome (intrauterine adhesions) will have a history of uterine instrumentation or pelvic tuberculosis, and the diagnosis can be confirmed with imaging such as sonohysterography, hysterosalpingography, or hysteroscopy. Patients with chronic anovulation or other endocrine disorders require additional workup accordingly.

DISPOSITION
Outpatient Care

Amenorrhea can be caused by different pathologies. Once the diagnosis is made, patient treatment can be individualized. As described earlier in this chapter, treatment can range from observation to medical management to surgical management.

WHAT YOU NEED TO REMEMBER

- Primary amenorrhea is characterized by no menses by age 14 to 16.
- Secondary amenorrhea is characterized by no menses for 6 months or three cycles for women who have previously had menstruation.
- The most common cause of amenorrhea is pregnancy.
- Three broad categories of amenorrhea are hypergonadotropic hypogonadism, hypogonadotropic hypogonadism, and eugonadism.
- The initial workup includes the measurement of history and physical exam findings, β-hCG, TSH, prolactin, FSH levels, and a progesterone withdrawal test.
- Patients with Turner syndrome (45 X,O) have gonads without follicles.
- You should remember to perform a gonadectomy in women with either Swyer syndrome or androgen resistance to reduce the risk of gonadal cancer.
- A constitutional delay of puberty is the most common cause of primary amenorrhea.
- Kallmann syndrome is associated with anosmia.
- Patients with müllerian agenesis can have renal, skeletal, and cardiac abnormalities.
- Patients with androgen resistance lack pubic hair on physical examination.

REFERENCE

1. Katz VL. Primary and secondary amenorrhea and precocious puberty: etiology, diagnostic evaluation, management. In: Katz VL, Lentz GM, Lobo RA, et al., eds. *Comprehensive Gynecology.* 5th ed. Philadelphia: Mosby; 2007.

SUGGESTED READINGS

Hickey M, Balen A. Menstrual disorders in adolescence: investigation and management. *Hum Reprod Update.* 2003;9:493–504.

Master-Hunter T, Heiman DL. Amenorrhea: evaluation and treatment. *Am Fam Physician.* 2006;73:1374–1382.

The Practice Committee of the American Society for Reproductive Medicine. Current evaluation of amenorrhea. *Fertil Steril.* 2006;86(Suppl 1):S148–S155.

Infertility

THE PATIENT ENCOUNTER

A 35-year-old woman (G0P0) and her husband see you in your clinic because of difficulty conceiving. The couple has been married for 5 years and has been actively trying to conceive without success. The female partner has never been pregnant. She reports irregular menses and an inability to predict her cycles. The male partner denies any complaints and has not fathered any children in the past. They request your assistance to conceive.

OVERVIEW

Definition

Fertility is defined as the ability to conceive and produce an offspring. Conversely, infertility is defined as the inability to conceive. Specifically, infertility is defined as an inability to conceive despite 12 months of frequent, unprotected intercourse. Because roughly 85% of couples will conceive within 1 year of attempting pregnancy, this leaves 15% of couples with the diagnosis of infertility. It is important to point out that the term *infertility* may be misleading in that it implies that the patient is either fertile or infertile. In fact, patients are more likely to be *sub*fertile rather than *in*fertile. This chapter will focus on how to evaluate the infertile couple and will discuss the treatment options available based on the diagnosis.

Pathophysiology

The pathophysiology of infertility is quite complex. It may be related to the female partner, the male partner, or both. Thus, an evaluation of both the male and the female is essential.

CLINICAL PEARL

Despite an adequate evaluation, roughly 10% of patients will fall under the category of unexplained infertility, in which a diagnosis is not reached. This lack of diagnosis can be very frustrating to both patients and their treating physicians.

Epidemiology

The prevalence of infertility has remained fairly stable since 1995 (1–3). Despite of this stability in prevalence, the incidence of primary infertility (women who have never conceived) has increased (2,3). This increased incidence in primary infertility may be attributed to several factors. The most notable of these factors includes a trend toward delayed childbearing and an increased incidence of sexually transmitted infections. Although in men, age does not affect fertility, there is an age-related decline in fertility in women. This decline in fertility is usually noted by age 35. For that reason, women who intentionally delay childbearing and who are close to reaching the age of 35 should be counseled on the age-related diminution of fertility. Also, sexually transmitted infections, such as chlamydia and gonorrhea, have the potential of damaging the female reproductive tract, specifically, the fallopian tubes.

Etiology

Many etiologic factors contribute to the diminished capacity of couples to conceive. Both the male and the female can contribute equally to infertility. As can be seen, female factors contribute roughly 60% to the diagnoses, while the male factors can contribute 40%. Although not depicted in the figure, it is not uncommon to discover a mixed picture during the evaluation in which both male and female factors contribute to the infertility.

CLINICAL PEARL

The two most common causes of female infertility are tubal disorders and ovulatory dysfunction.

Finally, it should be noted that there is a category of patients in whom a thorough evaluation will not render a diagnosis. These patients are categorized as having unexplained causes of infertility.

In order to achieve a successful pregnancy, the following conditions must be present:

1. The central nervous system (hypothalamus/pituitary) should send stimulating signals to the ovary (follicle-stimulating hormone [FSH]).
2. The ovary responds and ovulation takes place.
3. Sperm is available to fertilize the released oocyte.
4. A patent and normal female genital tract allows sperm to reach the oocyte and the resultant embryo to reach the endometrial cavity for implantation.

To be simplistic, for a successful pregnancy to occur, a functional central nervous system, a responsive ovary, patent fallopian tubes, and a normal semen analysis are required. Any perturbation at any of these steps can lead to infertility. The evaluation of an infertile couple is based on detecting abnormalities in these steps.

ACUTE MANAGEMENT AND WORKUP

It is important to point out that even though infertility is not considered a disease by many, it essentially is a disease. Although virtually all diagnoses stemming from infertility evaluations are not considered life-threatening, they *are* life-altering. Although there is usually no emergent need to work up and treat an infertile couple, a female patient that presents at or after the age of 35 will require expeditious evaluation and treatment because of the age-related diminution of fertility.

The First 15 Minutes

This time is usually spent by the couple in the outpatient setting. The couple may be asked to fill out a questionnaire in order to assist with the evaluation process. The questionnaire is usually directed at the patient's current problem and whether prior treatments were pursued. In addition, questions are included regarding general health and past medical problems.

Initial Assessment

The initial assessment takes place in the office setting. Both the male and the female patient are usually asked to be present for the initial assessment. During that time, a complete history of each person is elicited and a physical examination is performed. Further testing and referrals will then be based on clinical suspicion.

The First Few Hours

As you begin the evaluation of an infertile couple, one of the first facts you must appreciate is what the patient's expectations are. The reproductive goals of your patient will help dictate how aggressive you choose to be.

History

A thorough history will document the past experience with attempting to conceive, and your job will be to review all of the information at your disposal and determine which tests need to be ordered or repeated.

The Female Partner

A medical, surgical, and family history, as well as a history of medications, should be elicited. In addition, the following specific information should be obtained:

- The duration of infertility
- The patient's obstetric history, including the number of prior pregnancies and their outcome
- The patient's gynecologic history, including her age at menarche, her cycle length and duration, and any history of sexually transmitted diseases
- A history of prior surgeries, especially pelvic surgery and cervical procedures

The duration of infertility will suggest the prognosis of infertility as well as the likelihood of successful treatment. Unfortunately, a worse prognosis is seen with a longer duration of infertility. The patient's obstetric history may provide information regarding pregnancy wastage, genetic abnormalities, or anatomic defects of the reproductive tract. Menstrual abnormalities may suggest conditions such as anovulation. Also, a history of sexually transmitted infections may indicate conditions such as fallopian tube obstruction. A history of endometriosis or prior abdominal surgery may also suggest tubal disease. If the cervix was treated surgically, that may affect cervical mucous production, which plays an important role as a sperm reservoir, protecting sperm from the acidic vaginal secretions.

The Male Partner

As with the female partner, the male partner's medical, surgical, and family history as well as medication history should be elicited. In addition, the following specific history should be obtained:

- Prior pregnancies of the male's partner(s)
- Developmental history, such as cryptorchidism and pubertal development
- Medical conditions, such as diabetes
- Prior treatment with chemotherapeutic agents or radiation therapy
- The use of saunas and hot tubs
- Current medications, recreational drug use (such as marijuana), alcohol consumption, tobacco use, and anabolic steroid use

Patients with cryptorchidism have a roughly 80% fertility rate if the condition was unilateral, while patients with a history of bilateral cryptorchidism have a 50% chance of fertility (4). Diabetes and certain medications have the potential of causing impotence or other conditions such as retrograde ejaculation. Treatment with chemotherapeutic agents or pelvic radiation may cause irreversible damage to the testes, which affects both sperm and testosterone production. The use of saunas and hot tubs, and occupations that cause an elevation in scrotal temperature can have a negative effect on sperm production and motility (5,6). Anabolic steroid use also leads to infertility by negatively affecting sperm production.

Both Female and Male Partners

Sexual practices, and specifically the timing of intercourse relative to the menstrual cycle, are important. Usually, in a 28-day menstrual cycle, ovulation will occur on cycle day 14. As the oocyte only survives for roughly 18 to 24 hours after ovulation, it is important for sperm to be available in the genital tract at about the time of ovulation. Also, inquiring about lubricant use is important because lubricants can have a negative effect on sperm.

Physical Examination

The physical exam should be focused on the historical findings.

The Female Partner

In the female, the physical exam is usually focused on the following:

- The patient's body habitus, weight, and body mass index
- Evidence of androgen excess, such as acne, hirsutism, male hair pattern, or clitoromegaly
- A pelvic exam, looking for obvious abnormalities such as cervical and uterine abnormalities or pelvic masses

If warranted, the female partner should be referred to her obstetrician/gynecologist or to an infertility specialist for further examination.

The Male Partner

In the male, the physical exam is usually focused on the genital exam and should assess for the following:

- The degree of virilization
- Testicular volume and consistency
- The presence of a varicocele
- The presence of the vas deferens

If warranted, the male partner should be referred to his primary physician or to a urologist for further examination.

Labs and Tests to Consider

The laboratory tests and tests you should consider are geared toward identifying the primary cause of infertility in your couple. A uniform, step-wise approach to the infertility workup will ensure that you are efficient with the laboratory tests ordered so as not to waste your couple's reproductive time. The issue can be either female or male factor.

The Female Partner

The laboratory investigations used in the evaluation of an infertile female should include ovulation testing as well as testing of the levels of thyroid-stimulating hormone and prolactin.

Laboratory investigations that should be obtained based on clinical findings include ovarian reserve testing in patients older than age 35 and androgen testing in patients with evidence of androgen excess on examination.

In the initial evaluation of all infertile females, ovulation should be confirmed. Most patients with regular, predictable menstrual cycles are most likely ovulatory. Patients such as the one in the case previously described, are likely anovulatory. Confirmation of ovulation can be done via several methods:

- Measurement of basal body temperature
- Home urine testing of luteinizing hormone (LH) level
- Measurement of day 21 (luteal phase) progesterone level

The measurement of basal body temperature and home urine testing of the LH level are simple tests that can be done by the patient in the comfort of her home. A rise of 0.5°F to 1.0°F (approximately 0.3°C to 0.6°C) from the baseline temperature usually signifies ovulation, while a positive urine LH test usually signifies imminent ovulation. Progesterone level testing is a more invasive test that requires a blood draw in a laboratory. The principle behind this test is that progesterone levels will raise in the luteal phase of the menstrual cycle if a patient ovulates. In the past, endometrial biopsies were frequently used for the purpose of examining the endometrium for progesterone effects, but this procedure has been largely replaced by the method previously mentioned, which is less invasive.

It is also suggested that all infertile patients have their levels of prolactin and thyroid-stimulating hormone measured. Hyperprolactinemia and thyroid abnormalities can be a cause of infertility, especially if they cause irregular menses. The treatment of infertility in these cases will be directed at treating the underlying abnormal condition.

Patients older than the age of 35 should have ovarian reserve testing. The simplest of these tests is measure of follicular phase FSH level, usually performed on the third day of menses. This level is elevated in cases of diminished ovarian reserve and signifies declined fertility.

Patients with evidence of hyperandrogenism (androgen excess) on examination may have polycystic ovary syndrome (PCOS). PCOS is the most common cause of irregular cycles and hyperandrogenism in reproductive-aged women. It affects roughly 5% of this population. Because PCOS is a diagnosis of exclusion, other conditions that may mimic PCOS should be excluded. To exclude other conditions, patients suspected of having PCOS require an evaluation of their testosterone level in addition to a 17α-hydroxyprogesterone (17-OHP) level. Testosterone is usually slightly elevated in patients with PCOS. If there is a significant elevation in the testosterone level, this may signify an androgen-producing tumor of either ovarian or adrenal origin. An elevation of the 17-OHP level may signify the presence of a condition called adult-onset congenital adrenal hyperplasia. Subsequently, further testing to rule out these conditions is required.

Imaging. Confirmation of tubal patency is essential in the infertility evaluation. Hysterosalpingography is the most commonly used tool for this purpose. This procedure entails instilling a dye in the endometrial cavity and a radiograph indicates the shape of the endometrial cavity and the patency of both fallopian tubes.

Imaging of the pelvis by sonography can also be considered if there is suspicion of pelvic pathology on physical examination.

Surgery as a Diagnostic Tool. Prior to the extensive use of diagnostic techniques such as ultrasonography, laparoscopic evaluation of the infertile patient was widely used. Diagnostic laparoscopy is intended to evaluate the pelvic structures, including tubal patency. Because laparoscopic surgery is an invasive procedure and most of the necessary information to complete an evaluation can be obtained by the previously mentioned tests, laparoscopy is usually reserved for those patients who have suspected pelvic pathology or who have failed initial treatment. Diagnostic laparoscopy may also play a role in patients who are diagnosed as having unexplained infertility. It can also be used as a therapeutic tool in case pathology is discovered.

The Male Partner

The initial test in males is semen analysis. The World Health Organization published the following normal parameters for semen analysis (7);

- Volume, $\geq$2.0 mL
- Concentration, $\geq$20 million sperms per milliliter
- Motility, $\geq$50% motile sperm
- Morphology, $\geq$30% normal sperm shapes

Based on the semen analysis findings, further testing can be performed. If sperm parameters are abnormal, endocrine testing, such as measures of the levels of testosterone, FSH, LH and prolactin, may be necessary. At that point, the patient is likely to benefit from a referral to a male infertility specialist.

Treatment

Treatment is based on the diagnosis (Fig. 23-1).

Anovulatory Patients

In the anovulatory patient, the treatment is directed at restoring ovulation. Anovulation can be secondary to several etiologies:

Eugonadotropic Patients. Eugonadotropic anovulation is most commonly related to PCOS. Patients with this condition have abnormally functioning ovaries in which there is an excess of androgen production, but normal estrogen production.

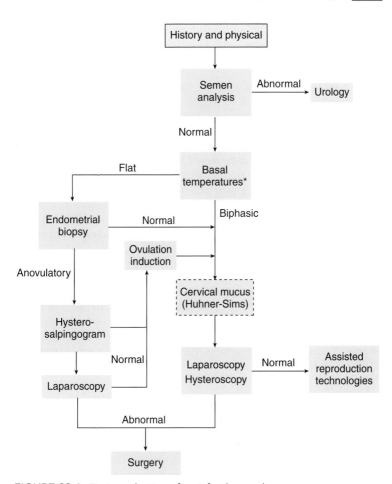

FIGURE 23-1: Basic evaluation of an infertile couple.

In the case of eugonadotropic anovulation, clomiphene citrate (Clomid) can be used. Clomid is a selective estrogen receptor modulator that is believed to act as a competitor with estrogen for the estrogen receptor at the level of the hypothalamus and pituitary. This action in turn leads to the release of gonadotropins from the pituitary gland, which stimulates ovarian follicle growth and eventually ovulation. The initial dose of Clomid is 50 mg daily given for 5 days starting on cycle day 3, 4, or 5 (cycle day 1 is the first day of full menstrual flow). Patients then test their urinary LH level at home in order to detect an LH surge or they undergo sonography in order to monitor follicular growth. Ovulation can also be artificially induced by administering an injection of human chorionic gonadotropin, which mimics the pituitary LH surge. Patients can then time intercourse to ovulation or an intrauterine insemination (IUI) can be performed.

If no follicular growth is seen, the Clomid dose is increased at the next cycle. However, certain patients remain resistant to the effects of Clomid and will require further treatment. In this case, either gonadotropin therapy or ovarian drilling is options that can be used. Ovarian drilling is a laparoscopic surgical procedure in which small punctures are made in both ovaries using either laser or unipolar cautery. This procedure is aimed at restoring ovulation. The alternative option, which is gonadotropin therapy, is an injectable FSH treatment aimed at directly stimulating ovarian follicle growth. Gonadotropins are available as urinary purified human menopausal gonadotropins or as a recombinant. Ovarian drilling and gonadotropin therapy have been reported to have equivalent pregnancy outcomes in patients resistant to Clomid (8).

Both treatments are not without complications. Ovarian drilling is a surgical procedure that carries both surgical and anesthetic risks. Gonadotropin therapy has a 25% risk of multiple gestations with 20% being twins and 5% being triplets or higher multiples. In addition to the risk of multiple gestations, ovarian hyperstimulation syndrome, which can be a life-threatening complication from ovarian stimulation, can develop in patients treated with gonadotropins. Patients not desiring either treatment or who have failed these treatments may decide to proceed to in vitro fertilization (IVF).

Patients with Hypergonadotropic Hypogonadism. These patients have primary ovarian failure and therefore their ovaries are not responsive to the normally produced LH and FSH from the pituitary gland. Depending on the severity of their condition, patients with primary ovarian failure may not respond to either Clomid or gonadotropin therapy. Treatment, even with IVF, usually renders poor results because the ovaries are no longer responsive to hormonal stimulation. The best option for these severe cases is either donor oocytes or adoption.

Patients with Hypogonadotropic Hypogonadism. These patients have hypothalamic or pituitary dysfunction that results from a lack of signaling from the central nervous system to the ovary. The ovaries are normal in these cases. Hyperprolactinemic patients also fall under this category.

Because of the mechanism of action of Clomid, patients with hypothalamic/pituitary dysfunction will not respond to this medication. These patients will benefit from gonadotropin therapy, which directly stimulates their ovaries. IVF is another valid treatment option.

Tubal Disease

The treatment of tubal disease includes surgical correction of the tubal pathology (tuboplasty) or IVF. The decision largely lies with the patient. Surgical correction is based on the extent of tubal damage. Severely damaged fallopian tubes may still remain nonfunctional even after surgical correction and may also cause harm by placing the patient at risk for future ectopic pregnancies. If the fallopian tubes are beyond repair, IVF is the better option. An attempt at tubal repair is not a prerequisite to proceeding with IVF. In fact, certain patients with repairable tubes prefer to proceed with IVF rather than surgery. It is recommended, though, that severe tubal pathology, such as hydrosalpinx, is removed prior to attempting IVF because tubal fluid efflux from abnormal tubes into the endometrial cavity can have a negative effect on a developing embryo and can therefore affect pregnancy rates (9). With the improvement of IVF pregnancy rates, careful counseling of the couple should be made. The cost of both treatments and their success rates should be presented to a couple so that this information can be factored into their decision.

In vitro fertilization, as the name implies, is fertilization of the oocyte outside the body, such as in a laboratory. Figure 23-2 depicts a sample treatment cycle for an IVF patient. The patient undergoes a series of injectable medications, which includes a gonadotropin (usually a recombinant FSH preparation). Once a cohort of follicles grows to an acceptable size, a human chorionic gonadotropin injection is given to cause final maturation of the developed oocytes, and then, under sonographic guidance, a needle is inserted transvaginally for oocyte collection (egg retrieval). The collected

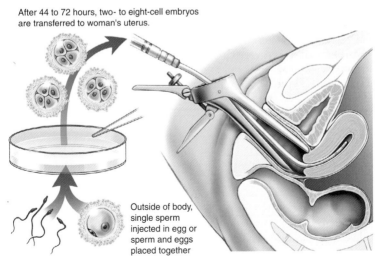

After 44 to 72 hours, two- to eight-cell embryos are transferred to woman's uterus.

Outside of body, single sperm injected in egg or sperm and eggs placed together

FIGURE 23-2: Sample n vitro fertilization treatment cycle.

oocytes are handed over to an embryologist who manages the fertilization process and follows the embryo progression. Once an embryo is formed, it is then transferred into the uterine cavity of the patient (embryo transfer).

Male Factor Infertility

If the semen parameters are slightly abnormal, this can be overcome by a procedure called intrauterine insemination. This procedure entails the collection of semen by masturbation. The andrology laboratory then processes the semen specimen and concentrates the sperm into a small volume to be directly instilled into the endometrial cavity. Severe sperm abnormalities in semen analysis should be evaluated by chromosomal analysis and hormonal evaluation of the male. For these evaluations, the patient is usually referred to a male infertility specialist.

In cases of significant low sperm counts, IVF with the addition of intracytoplasmic sperm injection (ICSI) has allowed many couples to conceive even with severely affected sperm numbers. During the ICSI procedure, one sperm is selected and directly injected into an oocyte by an embryologist in the embryology laboratory.

Finally, donated sperm should be considered as another option in couples with severe male-factor infertility. Similar to the use of the male partner's sperm, donor sperm can be used for IUI, IVF, and ICSI.

Unexplained Infertility

Because patients expect a diagnosis at the end of an evaluation, the lack of pathologic findings can be frustrating for them. Table 23-1 shows the

TABLE 23-1
Efficacy of Treatment for Unexplained Infertility

Treatment Type	Pregnancy Rate (%)
Control (No treatment)	1.3–4.1
IUI	3.8
Clomid	5.6
Clomid + IUI	8.3
HMG	7.7
HMG + IUI	17.1
IVF	20.7

IUI, intrauterine insemination; HMG, human menopausal gonadotropin; IVF, in vitro fertilization.

success rates of the different treatment options available for patients with unexplained infertility (10). Based on these data, it is safe to say that the minimum treatment should be Clomid with IUI. More aggressive treatment, such as gonadotropins or IVF, can also be considered based on the patients' desires. Of note, none of the treatments are a prerequisite for more advanced treatments.

For all types of diagnoses, adoption should be an option presented to all infertile couples. Most couples with infertility will initially desire treatment for their conditions and should consider adoption in the case of treatment failure. Couples interested in adoption should be referred to the proper individuals familiar with their state's adoption laws.

EXTENDED IN-HOSPITAL MANAGEMENT

In-hospital care is not usually required for infertility evaluation or management. It may only be required if the treatment is surgical in nature and requires a postoperative monitoring phase in the hospital.

DISPOSITION

Discharge Goals

After treatment, once a patient is found to be pregnant, the pregnancy is usually confirmed by serially following beta-human chorionic gonadotropin levels and confirmation by ultrasonography.

Outpatient Care

Many infertility specialists will monitor the pregnancy with serial ultrasound examinations until the patient gets through the first trimester (13 weeks). This is the time in pregnancy when the risk of spontaneous miscarriage is the highest. Obstetric care by a general obstetrician/gynecologist is then initiated.

WHAT YOU NEED TO REMEMBER

- Both men and women can contribute to infertility.
- Infertility is defined as an inability to conceive despite 12 months of frequent, unprotected intercourse.
- The two most common causes of female infertility are ovulatory disorders and tubal disorders.
- For a successful pregnancy to occur, a functional central nervous system, a responsive ovary (ovulation), patent fallopian tubes, and normal sperm are required.

- Initial evaluation of the infertile male includes semen analysis.
- Patients with primary ovarian failure may need to use donor oocytes to attain a successful pregnancy.
- Among the various treatment options for unexplained infertility, IVF provides the best pregnancy rates.

REFERENCES

1. Horn MC, Mosher WD. Use of services for family planning and infertility. United States, 1982. *Vital Health Stat 23.* 1986;(13):1–58.
2. Abma JC, Chandra A, Mosher WD, et al. Fertility, family planning, and women's health: new data from the 1995 National Survey of Family Growth. *Vital Health Stat 23.* 1997;(19):1–114.
3. Chandra A, Martinez GM, Mosher WD, et al. Fertility, family planning, and reproductive health of U.S. women: data from the 2002 National Survey of Family Growth. *Vital Health Stat 23.* 2005;(25):1–160.
4. Lee PA. Fertility in cryptorchidism: does treatment make a difference? *Endocrinol Metab Clin North Am.* 1993;22:479–490.
5. Saikhun J, Kitiyanant Y, Vanadurongwan V, et al. Effects of sauna on sperm movement characteristics of normal men measured by computer-assisted sperm analysis. *Int J Androl.* 1998;21:358–363.
6. Bujan L, Daudin M, Charlet JP, et al. Increase in scrotal temperature in car drivers. *Hum Reprod.* 2000;15:1355–1357.
7. World Health Organization. Reference values of semen variables. *WHO Laboratory Manual for the Examination of Human Semen and Sperm-Cervical Mucous Interaction.* New York: Cambridge University Press; 1999:60–61.
8. Farquhar C, Lilford RJ, Marjoribanks J, et al. Laparoscopic 'drilling' by diathermy or laser for ovulation induction in anovulatory polycystic ovary syndrome. *Cochrane Database Syst Rev* 2007;(3):CD001122.
9. Zeyneloglu HB, Arici A, Olive DL. Adverse effects of hydrosalpinx on pregnancy rates after in vitro fertilization-embryo transfer. *Fertil Steril.* 1998;70:492–499.
10. Guzick DS, Sullivan MW, Adamson GD, et al. Efficacy of treatment for unexplained infertility. *Fertil Steril.* 1998;70:207–213.

SUGGESTED READINGS

Carr BR, Blackwell RE, Azziz R. *Essential Reproductive Medicine.* New York: McGraw-Hill; 2005.
Consensus on infertility treatment related to polycystic ovary syndrome. *Fertil Steril.* 2008;89:505–522.
Forti G, Krausz C. Clinical review 100: evaluation and treatment of the infertile couple. *J Clin Endocrinol Metab.* 1998;83:4177–4188.
Speroff L, Fritz MA. *Clinical Gynecologic Endocrinology and Infertility.* 7th ed. Philadelphia: Lippincott Williams & Wilkins, 2005.

Perimenopause and Menopause

THE PATIENT ENCOUNTER

A 47-year-old woman (G3P3) presents to your clinic complaining of "hot flashes" and irregular bleeding for the past 12 months. The patient previously had regular menstrual cycles and reports weight gain, fatigue, and increasing irritability for the past few months.

OVERVIEW

Definition

Menopause is the clinical manifestation of ovarian failure characterized by the cessation of menstrual cycles. This transition from the reproductive to the nonreproductive phase of female biology is usually preceded by perimenopause, a stage during which many women experience menstrual irregularities as well as other systemic changes ranging from sexual dysfunction to cardiovascular disorders. Menopause is a process that is mediated primarily by a falling estradiol level but, most importantly, it is a very distressing period for many patients. This chapter will focus on the causes, effects, and management of perimenopause and menopause.

Pathophysiology

Through a little-understood mechanism, the number of follicles within the female ovary decreases throughout a woman's adult life and reaches its nadir at about the time of perimenopause. As the follicles are depleted, the levels of inhibin B and progesterone (produced by the granulosa cells of the developing follicles) fall and cause elevation of follicle-stimulating hormone (FSH) levels via a tightly regulated closed feedback loop. The increase in FSH will initially help maintain a normal level of estradiol until the time of complete ovarian failure (menopause) or the depletion of ovarian follicles. At this time, a woman will enter an estrogen-deficient state and may experience some of the following symptoms:

- Irregular bleeding
- Vasomotor symptoms
- Genitourinary symptoms
- Cardiovascular symptoms
- Musculoskeletal symptoms, including osteoporosis

- Psychiatric symptoms
- Other systemic symptoms

Epidemiology

The average age of menopause in the United States is 51 years. The median age of perimenopause is 47.5 years, with the median length being 4 years. As we see the world population continue to increase, the care of postmenopausal women will remain an important aspect of health care. Over the last 5 years, the number of people older than age 60 worldwide nearly doubled. The number of women entering menopause in the United States will nearly double from 1990 to 2020 (1,2).

Etiology

Menopause, defined as amenorrhea for 12 months, is a gradual, multiphase process that is best summarized by the stages of reproductive aging workshop (STRAW) in 2001 (Table 24-1). The STRAW system separates menopause into two phases: (i) the transitional phase, which is often characterized by menstrual irregularities and vasomotor symptoms, and (ii) postmenopause, which is defined by the absence of menstruation for 1 year.

It is interesting to note that the average age of menopause, 51 years, has remained relatively unchanged throughout the years. This is because, unlike

TABLE 24-1
Menopause Stages: the Stages of Reproductive Aging Workshop (STRAW) Staging System

Stages:	-5	-4	-3	-2	-1	0 Final menstrual period (FMP)	+1	+2
Terminology:	Reproductive			Menopausal transition			Postmenopause	
	Early	Peak	Late	Early	Late*		Early*	Late
				Perimenopause				
Duration of stage:	Variable			Variable		(a) 1 yr	(b) 4 yrs	until demise
Menstrual cycles:	Variable to regular	Regular		Variable cycle length (>7 days different from normal)	≥2 skipped cycles and an interval of amenorrhea (≥60 days)	Amen × 12 months	None	
Endocrine:	Normal FSH		↑ FSH	↑ FSH			↑ FSH	

*Stages most likely to be characterized by vasomotor symptoms.

puberty, environmental factors such as nutrition and body habitus play a minor role in the onset of menopause. Rather, menopause is a process that takes place as a result of a genetically programmed loss of ovarian follicles and the hormonal changes that take place thereafter. A few of the postulated factors that may predispose a woman to early menopause include:

- A family history of early menopause
- A history of diabetes mellitus type I
- Smoking
- The presence of variant form of galactose-1-phospate uridyl transferase

ACUTE MANAGEMENT AND WORKUP

The menopausal transition will rarely present with acute changes that warrant in-hospital evaluation. Nevertheless, the symptoms are usually unnerving and require an evaluation to confirm a normal transition.

The First 15 Minutes

The hormonal shift includes a slightly elevated level of estradiol combined with a progesterone deficiency and leads to an anovulatory environment, which results in irregular bleeding.

Initial Assessment

If the patient presents with a long-standing history of irregular vaginal bleeding, make sure to check her complete blood count to evaluate her levels of hemoglobin and hematocrit. It is not uncommon for perimenopausal women to present with an acute blood loss anemia that may require a blood transfusion.

Admission Criteria and Level of Care Criteria

The three conditions in which a menopausal patient needs to be admitted to the hospital are acute blood loss anemia, a pathologic bone fracture, and when the patient is suspected of having a major depressive disorder with suicidal and/or homicidal ideations.

The First Few Hours

Menopause management is commonly performed in an outpatient setting. The initial consultation with a physician will help prioritize the symptom constellation and aid with directing the appropriate therapy.

History

The workup of the common clinical manifestations of menopause includes an evaluation of irregular bleeding as well as vasomotor, genitourinary, cardiovascular, systemic, musculoskeletal, and psychiatric symptoms.

Irregular Bleeding

Relatively normal to slightly elevated level of estradiol combined with progesterone deficiency during the transition phase of menopause create an anovulatory environment that results in irregular vaginal bleeding. An endometrial biopsy or a transvaginal sonogram can be used to evaluate the endometrial stripe; an endometrial stripe <4 mm is less concerning for any endometrial pathology. Also consider a thyroid-stimulating hormone factor test to screen for any thyroid disease. It is important to carefully evaluate the cervix and the vaginal canal for any infections (cervicitis, sexually transmitted disease) or abnormal lesions (cervical polyps, cancer). The patient may benefit from oral contraceptive pills to regulate her menses or cyclic progesterone to empty her endometrial lining. It is crucial for patients to understand that cyclic progesterone will not provide contraception.

CLINICAL PEARL

For any woman older than 35 years of age, it is important to evaluate any complaint of irregular menses carefully to rule out endometrial hyperplasia or cancer.

Vasomotor Symptoms

The initial workup of a patient who presents with complaints of hot flashes must always include a carefully obtained history and a laboratory workup to exclude other causes. Some disease processes that may present similarly to perimenopause and menopause include tuberculosis (especially with known exposure, night sweats, and cough), lymphoma, and hypothyroidism and hyperthyroidism. Of the 75% of the women who experience hot flash symptoms, only 20% seek medical attention. Hot flashes are a process due to changes in the hypothalamic thermoregulation by the shifting estrogen level. It is often described as sudden generalized body heat sensation that lasts seconds to minutes and is often accompanied by palpitations, perspiration, and/or anxiety. The onset is often unpredictable but is more common at night, making insomnia a common complaint among women in the menopausal age group. Hot flashes are often self-limited but if the symptoms are severe and interfere with the quality of life, medical therapy with antidepressants or estrogen (the gold standard) may be indicated.

Genitourinary Symptoms

Genitourinary symptoms include vaginal symptoms, sexual dysfunction, and urinary symptoms.

Vaginal Symptoms. The vaginal tissue is extremely estrogen-responsive and a decreased level of estrogen leads to atrophy. This atrophy causes vaginal dryness, vaginal itching, dyspareunia, and increased vaginal infections. A careful examination is warranted to rule out any organic causes and the patient may benefit from either systemic or topical estrogen.

Symptoms of Sexual Dysfunction. Causes are mechanical as well as systemic; as the level of estrogen falls, the amount of vasculature to the vagina diminishes, which results in less lubrication during intercourse. The length and the size of the vaginal canal may decrease secondary to vaginal atrophy, contributing to sexual discomfort. Recommend a short course of estrogen therapy and continued intercourse to prevent vaginal shortening.

Urinary Symptoms. As estrogen level falls, the pH of the vaginal canal becomes more basic, from <4.5 to 6.0. This shift in the pH alters the vaginal flora and may predispose a patient to more frequent urinary tract infections. Check a urinalysis and a urine culture if a patient complains of dysuria and/or urinary frequency. Treat any infection as indicated along with a short course of topical or systemic estrogen to normalize the pH of the vaginal canal and, thus, the flora of the vagina.

Cardiovascular Symptoms

Fortunately, the much-publicized increased risk of cardiovascular disease during menopause is limited to women over the age of 65. The use of exogenous estrogen has shown to reduce mortality from cardiovascular disease because it has a direct effect on arterial walls and it also has benign effects on the cholesterol profile (an increase in high-density lipoprotein and a decrease in low-density lipoprotein). However, the use of estrogen for the primary prevention of cardiac disease is not currently recommended by the American Heart Association.

Systemic Symptoms

Systemic symptoms include dementia and headaches.

Dementia. In literature, estrogen has been shown to lessen the incidences of dementia. It is important for a physician to distinguish dementia (nonreversible) from delirium (usually reversible). Alzheimer dementia is the most common form of dementia, but you should consider other causes, such as vascular dementia.

Headaches. Headache is one of the most common complaints during menopause; studies have shown that migraine headaches tend to lessen after menopause, whereas tension headaches worsen after menopause. It is of utmost importance, however, to perform a complete physical exam, including a neurologic exam, and rule out any organic causes in all patients who present complaining of headaches of acute onset. Computed tomography scans and magnetic resonance imaging can be ordered as indicated by the physical exam.

Musculoskeletal Symptoms

Some studies have shown an increase in the incidences of arthritis during the transition stage of menopause. Because the elderly population is especially at a higher risk of osteoporosis, exclude fractures or any recent history of fall or trauma. Plain radiographic films can be considered as a first-line test to evaluate any bone or joint pain.

There is an increased rate of bone reabsorption during menopause, especially in the first 5 years of onset. A DEXA bone scan may be indicated to evaluate bone density, especially in high-risk groups, such as whites, Asians, and patients with a family history of osteoporosis and dementia. Exogenous estrogen is no longer considered as the first-line treatment of osteoporosis. Currently, bisphosphates (alendronate) are the preferred first-line treatment.

Psychiatric Symptoms

Women with a history of depression and/or premenstrual syndrome symptoms are at an increased risk for depressive/mood disorders during menopause. However, a physician should keep in mind that depressive symptoms may not be related to hormonal changes but to other life stressors or environmental factors. Be sure to ask patients about the symptoms of major depressive disorder, including suicidal ideation, insomnia, guilt, changes in energy or appetite, an inability to concentrate, and psychomotor symptoms. A positive screen results in two of the aforementioned symptoms for >6 month duration.

Labs and Tests to Consider

Using all the symptom information previously presented, the key laboratory evaluations and tests to consider as you initiate care in a menopausal patient include the following:

- Endometrial biopsy
- Thyroid-stimulating hormone level
- Luteinizing hormone level
- FSH
- Vaginal pH
- Urinalysis
- DEXA scan

Treatment

After the recent reports from the Women's Health Initiative trials, the use of hormone-replacement therapy has dramatically decreased by many primary care providers. Depending on the symptoms ailing the patient, postmenopausal hormone therapy is still reasonable and recommended for short-term use.

Estrogen is available in many different preparations: topical, oral, and transdermal (transdermal presents the lowest risk of venous thrombosis). Physiological replacement doses include 0.625 mg of conjugated equine estrogen, 0.5 mg of micronized estradiol, or 0.05 mg of transdermal estradiol daily.

Although estrogen has many associated benefits, it should not be used in the following patient groups:

- Women with a history of breast cancer
- Women with a history of previous venous thrombotic events
- Women who have had strokes
- Patients who seek to prevent heart disease and osteoporosis

Unopposed estrogen should not be used in patients with a uterus as it will promote endometrial hyperplasia and cancer. A patient should get regular mammograms to rule out any breast pathologies. Women who have already had a hysterectomy do not need progestin therapy added to their estrogen.

A few simple rules of thumb regarding hormone replace therapy include the following:

- Use the lowest dose of estrogen with or without progesterone necessary to relive the primary symptoms.
- Initiate the therapy as close to menopause as possible.
- Use the hormones for a short amount of time (3 to 5 years).

EXTENDED IN-HOSPITAL MANAGEMENT

Rarely is in-hospital management for menopause indicated. If a patient is admitted for acute blood loss anemia, the physician should always make sure that a patient's vital signs are within normal limits and the patient should be transfused as necessary. Many times, additional estrogen therapy is necessary to stabilize the endometrium and help avert the acute bleeding.

DISPOSITION

Discharge Goals

After stabilizing the patient's symptoms, outpatient hormone therapy should be initiated until the patient has had a chance to fully recover. In the setting of vaginal bleeding, estrogen should be followed by cyclic progesterone to avoid the development of endometrial hyperplasia.

Outpatient Care

Regular clinic visits should occur every 6 months until the proper dose of hormones has been achieved. After 1 to 2 years, attempts can be made to wean the patient off hormone-replacement therapy. It is very important to continue breast and cervical cancer surveillance during the patient's annual evaluations.

WHAT YOU NEED TO REMEMBER

- Menopause is defined by a period of amenorrhea for 12 months.
- Menopause is a genetically programmed loss of ovarian follicles that results in decreased inhibin, an increased FSH level, and a diminished estrogen level.
- The loss of estrogen has many consequences, including genitourinary atrophy. Common complaints include vasomotor symptoms and irregular vaginal bleeding during transitional menopause.
- Exogenous estrogen is the gold standard of the treatment of vasomotor symptoms but should not be used in women with an increased risk of venous thrombosis, a history of strokes, or a history of breast cancer.
- Only short-term estrogen use is recommended (3 to 5 years) in patients. However, it is no longer recommended for the prevention of cardiovascular disease or for the treatment of osteoporosis.

REFERENCES

1. North American Menopause Society. Section A: Overview of menopause and aging. In: *Menopause Practice: A Clinicians Guide.* Cleveland, OH: Author; 2004.
2. Katz VL, Lentz GM, Lobo RA, et al. *Comprehensive Gynecology.* 5th ed. Philadelphia: Mosby; 2007.

SUGGESTED READINGS

Casper RF, Barbieri RL, Crowley WF, et al. Clinical manifestations and diagnosis of menopause. Available at: http://www.uptodate.com. Version 16.1, 2006. Accessed November 19, 2008.

Martin KA, Barbieri RL, Crowley WF, et al. Treatment of menopausal symptoms with hormone therapy. Available at: http://www.uptodate.com. Version 16.1, 2007. Accessed November 19, 2008.

Welt CK, Barbieri RL, Crowley WF, et al. Ovarian development and failure (menopause) in normal women. Available at: http://www.uptodate.com. Version 16.1, 2007. Accessed November 19, 2008.

Pelvic Relaxation

THE PATIENT ENCOUNTER

A 56-year-old woman (G4P4) presents to your clinic with pelvic fullness and difficulty urinating. She reports a dragging sensation in her pelvis that is worse in the evenings and that has become gradually more severe over the past year. She also reports dysuria with frequency, urgency, and the feeling that her bladder is still full after urination. She has an occasional leakage of urine with vigorous exercise and in the past few weeks has noticed a lump in her vagina after voiding.

OVERVIEW

Definition

Pelvic relaxation, or prolapse, occurs with the descent of one or more pelvic structures into the vaginal canal. Anterior wall relaxation typically involves the bladder (cystocele) with or without coexistent urethral prolapse (cystourethrocele). Apical defects result in prolapse of the uterus, or, after hysterectomy, of the vaginal cuff. Posterior wall relaxation includes herniation of the rectum (rectocele), the small bowel (enterocele), or the sigmoid colon (sigmoidocele) (1). This chapter will focus on the risk factors, evaluation, and management of pelvic organ prolapse.

Pathophysiology

The pelvic floor muscles are the primary support for the pelvic organs; they provide a flexible yet strong platform to counteract intra-abdominal and gravitational forces. The visceral connective tissues, or endopelvic fascia, and their thickenings form ligaments that stabilize the pelvic organs in position on this muscular base. With pelvic muscle weakness, increasing stress on endopelvic fascial attachments causes breaks, stretching, or attenuation of these supports, resulting in prolapse of the affected organs (1).

Epidemiology

As the population ages and life expectancy increases, pelvic relaxation will be encountered with greater frequency. Approximately 2% to 3% of women have significant pelvic support defects (2). The lifetime risk of undergoing corrective surgery for pelvic organ prolapse is 11%, and it is the most common indication for hysterectomy in women older than age 55 (3,4).

Etiology

Vaginal delivery of a term infant is postulated to be the most significant factor involved in the development of pelvic organ prolapse, but previous surgery to correct prolapse is the single greatest risk factor for *severe* prolapse when the various risk factors are analyzed (2). Other possible risk factors include genetic predisposition, parity, menopause, advancing age, prior pelvic surgery, connective tissue disorders, diabetes, pulmonary disease, factors associated with elevated intraabdominal pressure, lifestyle factors, and race (2,5).

CLINICAL PEARL

The various risk factors can be remembered with the mnemonic PROLAPSED:

Predisposition (genetic)
Race
Other (connective tissue disease, diabetes mellitus, pulmonary disease)
Lifestyle factors (smoking, obesity, high-impact sports)
Advancing age
Parity, postmenopausal
Surgery for prolapse
Elevated intra-abdominal pressure (chronic constipation, chronic cough, obesity)
Delivery of a term infant

ACUTE MANAGEMENT AND WORKUP

Pelvic relaxation is typically managed as an outpatient condition, but complications related to the prolapse may prompt emergency department visits. Common reasons for acute presentation include urinary tract infection from obstruction and urinary stasis, bleeding and discharge from mucosal ulceration, urinary retention following incontinence surgery, or pelvic pain. Life-threatening ureteral obstruction, sepsis, and incarceration are rare (6).

The First 15 Minutes

Whether the patient is seen in the emergency department or the clinic, the initial assessment should focus on excluding acute complications, especially if the patient appears ill. As previously noted, life-threatening complications are uncommon, and the patient may have developed compensatory mechanisms such as digital reduction to effect symptom relief by facilitating urination, defecation, or by simply causing disappearance of the protruding mass (1). The initial assessment should be brief and focused.

Initial Assessment

The initial assessment includes eliciting a brief history, observing the patient, monitoring key vital signs, and performing a pelvic exam.

- History
  - Acute pain with an inability to urinate suggests acute retention.
  - Dysuria with fevers suggests cystitis; concomitant flank pain may indicate upper urinary tract involvement.
- Patient observation
  - Disorientation, mental status changes, or an ill-appearing patient suggests systemic infection or sepsis.
  - Severe pain suggests acute urinary retention or pyelonephritis from reflux or ureteral obstruction.
- Vital signs
  - An elevated temperature and heart rate suggest infection.
- Pelvic examination
  - Mucosal ulceration of prolapse with induration and erythema suggests infection while irreducibility may signal impending incarceration.

Admission Criteria and Level of Care Criteria

For life-threatening complications, admission with appropriate management is necessary. Transurethral catheterization for acute urinary retention and antibiotics for uncomplicated urinary tract infections with outpatient management is usually appropriate.

The First Few Hours

The initial assessment serves to triage patients into two groups: (i) patients who need inpatient admission for severe complications, and (ii) patients who can be treated and managed safely as outpatients. The latter group accounts for the majority of these patients.

History

The most specific symptom of prolapse is seeing or feeling a bulge protruding from the vagina. However, the finding of prolapse on exam does not correlate well with specific symptoms (5). Thus, the degree to which a patient is bothered by her symptoms is probably the most important consideration to guide management decisions. A detailed history of pain or discomfort should be taken, and direct questioning about symptoms related to urinary, defecatory, and sexual function and dysfunction must be included for a thorough evaluation. A number of validated questionnaires are available to assess symptom severity and quality of life issues (1).

> ### CLINICAL PEARL
>
> *Most women with pelvic relaxation are asymptomatic or will not report symptoms because of embarrassment.*

Physical Examination

The pelvic exam is of paramount importance for the evaluation of pelvic support defects. After a general abdominal exam, inspection of the external genitalia and a bimanual exam should be performed as up to two thirds of patients have coexistent gynecologic pathology (1). With the patient resting in the dorsal lithotomy position, a Sims retractor or the posterior blade of a bivalve speculum is used to retract the vaginal walls and evaluate the extent of the prolapsed parts. The exam should be performed in both a resting state and while straining to appreciate the full extent of the prolapse. The Pelvic Organ Prolapse Quantification Classification System, or POP-Q, evaluates prolapse by measuring a number of specific points relative to the hymen and should be performed in all women with pelvic relaxation (1). A Q-tip test for urethral hypermobility may be useful to evaluate incontinent patients who may benefit from surgical elevation of the bladder neck (2), and a rectovaginal exam is useful for assessment of posterior defects and fecal impaction. The neurologic exam should include an assessment of pelvic floor muscles, sensory testing, and an evaluation of sphincter function (1).

Labs and Tests to Consider

A careful history and physical exam are usually sufficient for diagnosing pelvic organ prolapse. All patients should have a urinalysis and post-void residual test. Ancillary tests may be needed to further evaluate voiding or defecatory dysfunction, as noted in the next section.

Key Diagnostic Labs and Tests

Pelvic relaxation is diagnosed mainly by history and physical exam. However, the following tests should be considered for patients with altered urinary or defecatory function:

1. *Urinalysis, Culture and Sensitivity.* These tests identify frank urinary tract infection in patients with irritative voiding symptoms, pelvic pain, or incontinence, as well as occult infection in patients with severe prolapse.
2. *Post-Void Residual.* In this test, the patient voids a measured amount and then undergoes catheterization for the amount remaining in the bladder. This test is useful for identifying patients with overflow incontinence and chronic urinary retention.

3. *Simple Cystometry.* During this test, a catheter is placed into the bladder and a 60-mL syringe barrel is attached. The bladder is filled slowly, allowing measurement of bladder capacity and bladder muscle contraction.

4. *Cough Stress Test.* During this test, the patient stands with a full bladder and coughs. Urinary leakage is considered a positive result.

5. *Multichannel Urodynamics.* This test involves the placement of transducers into the bladder and rectum to measure intravesical and intra-abdominal pressures, respectively. This testing can identify occult incontinence or can help to differentiate an overactive bladder from stress urinary incontinence.

6. *Defecatory Dysfunction.* Tests to evaluate defecatory dysfunction include anoscopy/proctosigmoidoscopy, colonic transit studies, and defecography.

Imaging

Because preoperative clinical assessments often do not correspond with intraoperative findings, imaging studies such as sonography and magnetic resonance imaging have been advocated to describe the exact nature of support defects. However, a lack of standardized criteria and unknown clinical utility currently limit widespread acceptance; thus, they are used mainly for research purposes (1).

Treatment

For the treatment of pelvic relaxation, a number of surgical and nonsurgical options exist. The choice of therapy is based on a number of factors, including the patient's baseline well-being (or ability to safely tolerate surgery), the patient's experiences with previous forms of therapy, and the patient's long-term expectations. In general, you should try some nonsurgical treatments before resorting to a major operative procedure.

Nonsurgical Management

Conservative Therapy. Generally appropriate for mild degrees of pelvic relaxation, symptom-directed therapy includes weight loss, smoking cessation, pelvic floor therapy (Kegel exercises), and optimal disease control (asthma, diabetes mellitus). For problems related to defecation, dietary modification, laxatives, and behavior training may aid in relieving symptoms, whereas timed voiding and an alteration of fluid intake may assist with symptoms of urinary incontinence (5).

Estrogen Therapy. The role of estrogen in pelvic relaxation is poorly understood. Currently, there are no data to support its use for the prevention or treatment of prolapse. However, estrogen should be used to treat mucosal ulceration and symptoms of urogenital atrophy, concomitantly with pessaries, and to optimize urogenital tissue health prior to surgical intervention (1).

Pessaries. Pessaries are inert silicone or plastic devices that are considered first-line therapy for the treatment of pelvic organ prolapse (5). They provide support by creating a functional obstruction in the vagina; some provide additional support to the bladder neck. Indications include pregnancy, contraindications to surgery, and whenever patient preference for a nonsurgical alternative exists. Pessaries can be fitted in any stage of prolapse and are not contraindicated in sexually active women.

Surgical Management

Apical Compartment. Abdominal or laparoscopic sacral colpopexy involves fixation of the vaginal apex to the sacrum, usually with synthetic mesh material. Transvaginal procedures such as sacrospinous or uterosacral ligament suspension use pelvic structures for fixation. Colpocleisis involves obliteration of the vagina by suturing a segment of the anterior vaginal wall to the posterior vaginal wall. It is suitable for women who do not desire vaginal function and who are at high risk of complications or who prefer to avoid hysterectomy (5).

Anterior Compartment. Anterior colporrhaphy reapproximates the pubocervical fascia in the midline with or without a graft. Paravaginal repair by a vaginal, retropubic, or laparoscopic approach serves to reattach the paravaginal tissues to endopelvic fascia overlying the obturator internus muscle.

Posterior Compartment. Posterior colporrhaphy is a midline plication of subepithelial vaginal tissue overlying the rectum.

Incontinence. Prophylactic anti-incontinence procedures should be considered concomitantly for severe stages of prolapse due to higher rates of postoperative stress urinary incontinence after repair (5).

EXTENDED IN-HOSPITAL MANAGEMENT

Pessaries are an indispensable tool for pelvic organ prolapse as they can be used to relieve short-term or long-term symptoms. Surgery for pelvic relaxation has a significant recurrence rate over time and carries significant risk of surgical complications (2). Failure rates for apical, anterior, and posterior wall prolapse procedures range from 0% to 20%, 15% to 37%, and 14% to 33%, respectively (5).

DISPOSITION

Discharge Goals

Patients admitted following surgery should meet the same discharge criteria as any postoperative patient. Postoperative pain should be controlled adequately with oral medications, and the patient should be able to tolerate oral intake with some recovery of bowel and bladder function. In addition, the patient should be afebrile and able to ambulate or mobilize independently without symptoms of dizziness. If an anti-incontinence procedure is performed, a voiding trial may be performed and the catheter removed before discharge, if successful.

Outpatient Care

With pessaries, the patient should return in 1 to 2 days after fitting and then at 4 to 6 weeks. After this initial follow-up, visits can be extended up to 6- to 12-month intervals, depending on the patient's ability to insert, remove, and clean it (1). The surveillance of postoperative patients for recurrence is mandatory. Visit intervals vary on the type and number of procedures and patient factors related to recurrence. Recurrence can be treated by repeat surgical procedures or consideration of alternate management strategies.

WHAT YOU NEED TO REMEMBER

- Most women with pelvic relaxation are asymptomatic.
- The degree to which a patient is bothered by her symptoms is probably the most important consideration to guide management decisions.
- Vaginal delivery of a term infant and previous surgery to correct prolapse are the most significant factors involved in the development of pelvic organ prolapse.
- In patients with pelvic organ prolapse, voiding, defecatory, and sexual dysfunction should be addressed.
- The patient history and physical exam are the key components in diagnosing pelvic relaxation.
- Management should aim to control symptoms in the least invasive manner.
- Pessaries are first-line management tools for pelvic organ prolapse.

REFERENCES

1. Walters MD, Karram MM. *Urogynecology and Reconstructive Pelvic Surgery.* 3rd ed. Philadelphia: Mosby; 2007.
2. Bent AE, Ostergard DR, Cundiff GW, et al., eds. *Ostergard's Urogynecology and Pelvic Floor Dysfunction.* 5th ed. Philadelphia: Lippincott Williams & Wilkins; 2003.

3. Olsen AL, Smith VJ, Bergstrom JO, et al. Epidemiology of surgically managed pelvic organ prolapse and urinary incontinence. *Obstet Gynecol.* 1997;89:501–506.
4. Wilcox LS, Koonin LM, Pokras R, et al. Hysterectomy in the United States, 1988-1990. *Obstet Gynecol.* 1994;83:549–555.
5. American College of Obstetricians and Gynecologists. ACOG practice bulletin number 85: pelvic organ prolapse. *Obstet Gynecol.* 2007;110:717–729.
6. American College of Obstetricians and Gynecologists. Precis: an update in obstetrics and gynecology. In: *Gynecology.* 2nd ed. Washington, DC: Author; 2006:54–73.

Urinary Incontinence

THE PATIENT ENCOUNTER

A 54-year-old patient (G5P4014) comes to your office for her annual physical examination. She underwent a hysterectomy with removal of both ovaries 4 years earlier because of a history of heavy and painful menses. She stopped taking hormone replacement within the last year, and now her only complaint is worsening urinary leakage. She had rare leakage over the last 10 years when she coughed or laughed with a full bladder, but now she is bothered by needing to urinate frequently during the day and night with loss of large volumes of urine when she gets a sudden, uncontrollable urge to void.

OVERVIEW

Definition

Urinary incontinence (UI) is the complaint of any involuntary leakage of urine (1).

Pathophysiology

The physiologic processes of bladder filling for urine storage interspersed with periods of efficient bladder emptying require complicated neural control of the bladder wall smooth muscle and the bladder outlet (internal and external urethral sphincters). A neural defect anywhere from the cerebral cortex to the bladder may result in bladder dysfunction. In addition, loss of anatomic support to the bladder base and urethra or surrounding connective tissue that results from obstetric trauma or the combined effects of aging, menopause, and other factors may affect the ability to maintain urine continence.

Epidemiology

Urinary incontinence is a common problem, occurring in approximately 25% of premenopausal women and 40% of postmenopausal women. Although not always bothersome, 10% of middle-aged women report daily UI and one-third report at least weekly UI (2). These rates are higher among nursing home patients. Because of patients' assumption that it is a normal part of aging or embarrassment on the part of the patient and sometimes the physician, UI is often underreported.

> ## CLINICAL PEARL
>
> *Urinary incontinence is very common and is underreported. Its incidence increases with age and with increasing degrees of pelvic relaxation.*

Etiology

The two most common forms of UI are stress and urge UI (SUI and UUI, respectively). Stress urinary incontinence is the involuntary leakage of urine with exertion, sneezing, or coughing that occurs when bladder pressure exceeds urethral resistance. This balance of pressures is influenced by intrinsic factors (urethral musculature, blood flow, and innervation) and extrinsic factors (the degree of urethral support, and the weight and physical activity of the patient) (3). Urge urinary incontinence is the involuntary leakage of urine accompanied by or immediately following a strong urge to urinate. In this case, involuntary and uninhibited bladder contractions (known as detrusor overactivity) overcome urethral resistance (3).

Anatomic abnormalities of the lower urinary tract may also cause UI. These include a fistulous tract from the bladder to the vagina or a diverticulum in the urethral wall. In the United States, fistulas usually result as a complication of pelvic surgery or pelvic radiation, and patients present with continuous leakage. Urethral diverticula are characterized by complaints of dribbling leakage of urine with position changes, dyspareunia, and dysuria related to frequent infections and chronic inflammation due to the pooling and stasis of urine within the diverticulum.

Overflow incontinence is the leakage of urine due to poor or absent bladder contractions leading to urinary retention, overdistention of the bladder, and incomplete emptying. Causes vary widely and include fecal impaction, medication side effects, and neurologic problems, such as lower motor neuron disease, autonomic neuropathy (diabetes), spinal cord injury, and multiple sclerosis.

- Finally, reversible and transient causes of urine leakage should be treated, when present, to potentially improve or alleviate UI symptoms. They are summarized using the mnemonic *DIAPPERS* (4):
  - **D**elirium—Treating reversible causes of patient confusion (such as medication side effects) may abate UI.
  - **I**nfection—Elderly women with urinary tract infection may present with UI as their only symptom.
  - **A**trophic vaginitis is associated with worsening urinary frequency, urgency, nocturia, and infection. Treat with local estrogen cream.
  - **P**harmacologic—Any medication with effects on the autonomic nervous system may influence lower urinary tract function; these

include cold medications, antihistamines, decongestants, and commonly prescribed antidepressants, sedative-hypnotics, and antihypertensives. The alpha-adrenergic blockers (e.g., prazosin, terazosin, doxazosin), in particular, may cause incontinence, while diuretics may aggravate existing UI.

- **P**sychological—Profoundly depressed patients may not care about maintaining continence, and UI can sometimes be used to gain attention or to manipulate others.
- **E**ndocrine—Causes include diabetes mellitus, diabetes insipidus, and hypercalcemia.
- **R**estricted mobility, such as after hip fracture, may make it impossible to reach a restroom in time to avoid an accident. Provide a bedside commode.
- **S**tool impaction in immobile patients may cause compression of the bladder and exacerbate other forms of incontinence.

ACUTE MANAGEMENT AND WORKUP

Patients with UI present with varied descriptions of what causes them to leak and with various degrees of anxiety over the condition. There is also heterogeneity in the amount of time a woman endures UI before presenting for treatment, but this is generally not an acute condition. Although a complete history is the important first step in the evaluation of a woman with UI, it is a poor predictor of the type of incontinence. Therefore, you should begin the general assessment with both a history and some form of objective investigation (4).

The First 15 Minutes

When a patient first presents for the evaluation of UI, you should carefully identify whether any transient conditions may be contributing to or causing the patient's complaint (see the mnemonic presented earlier).

Initial Assessment

As the patient enters the clinic, it is helpful to acquire a clean-catch midstream urine specimen to check with an office dipstick and subsequently with laboratory urine analysis and culture. This allows you to assess for urinary tract infection and possibly glucosuria from poorly controlled diabetes as potential contributors to UI. The voided volume is documented and then a post-void residual (PVR) is checked either by ultrasound scanner or by in-and-out bladder catheterization. Consensus seems to exist that a PVR of <50 to 100 mL is normal and >200 mL is abnormal (4). An elevated PVR may be found in a patient with overflow incontinence or from urinary retention due to urethral obstruction from a bulging cystocele or prior pelvic surgery.

The First Few Hours

Once the urine specimen, voided volume, and PVR have been documented and assessed, the initial evaluation of the incontinent patient may proceed.

History

A comprehensive history begins with flushing out the details of the chief complaint related to UI. This should include the duration and characteristics of the incontinent episodes, the frequency of UI, the use of protective devices, previous therapy, and any conditions that may predispose the patient to UI. It is helpful to document if the patient has leakage during stress events such as cough and sneeze, exercise, with intercourse or orgasm, and whether unconscious leakage occurs. Irritative voiding symptoms such as frequency, urgency, and dysuria need be documented. Recurrent or recent urinary infection or hematuria should be noted, as should symptoms that may be related to pelvic organ prolapse, including the need to splint to urinate by pushing down on the abdomen, changing positions on the commode, pushing up a vaginal bulge, or needing to perform a Valsalva maneuver in order to urinate. A sensation of incomplete emptying or the need to wait for a post-void dribble may also signal a cystocele or other prolapse as a contributing problem to the UI. Importantly, it is necessary to assess the patient's degree of bother by her UI symptoms; the presence of UI does not always necessitate treatment.

A complete past medical and surgical history is required. The social history will likely include alcohol and tobacco use, as smoking may result in a chronic cough and diminished blood flow with weakened connective tissue supports and worsening SUI. Alcohol, tobacco products, caffeine, and acidic foods and beverages are common bladder wall irritants that may contribute to detrusor contractions and UUI. Many drugs, as discussed previously, may cause or contribute to worsening UI symptoms, so it is important to list all prescribed and over-the-counter medications. The obstetric history should record the route of delivery, the weight of the largest child, and any other significant event such as forceps-assisted delivery and episiotomy or perineal lacerations.

Physical Examination

The initial exam begins with a general observation of mobility, cognitive status, peripheral edema, and body habitus. The abdominal exam includes documenting the location of previous surgical scars and assessing for suprapubic tenderness and obvious abdominopelvic masses or ascites. Patients should undergo a thorough neurologic examination. This consists of testing lower extremity deep tendon reflexes, anal reflex, the strength of pelvic floor contraction on bimanual examination, and the bulbocavernosus reflex, which can be seen as a twitch of the muscles around the vestibule with gentle stroking of the labia majora with the wooden end of a cotton swab.

The pelvic exam is central to the evaluation. The presence of a pool of urine in the vagina suggests a fistula, and a tender discrete mass of the anterior vaginal wall may indicate a urethral diverticulum. The degree of vaginal atrophy is documented. An assessment should be made of the degree of any pelvic organ prolapse using a Sims or disarticulated Graves speculum to retract the posterior or anterior vaginal walls while the patient is straining. A supine and/or standing cough stress test is performed by having the patient cough and perform a Valsalva maneuver with a full bladder to watch for urine leakage. A cotton swab test may be performed to assess the degree of urethral mobility.

CLINICAL PEARL

The urethra is deemed "hypermobile" if the lubricated sterile swab in the urethra and bladder deviates more than 30 degrees from the horizontal.

Labs and Tests to Consider

As previously discussed, it is appropriate to order a urinalysis plus a urine culture and to check the patient's PVR. If the history suggests an endocrinologic source of UI, blood chemistries and electrolyte levels may be considered to assess for diabetes or hypercalcemia.

A voiding diary can be a very helpful adjunct to the patient's history and physical exam. The diary consists of a list of patient intake and output over a 3- to 7-day period. The frequency of urinary episodes, the volume voided, and the timing of leakage events are documented. Ideally, the patient records the type of intake (e.g., coffee and tea, which are common bladder irritants) and what event precipitated urine leakage (e.g., a strong cough). The diary helps to objectively quantify nocturia, as well as the frequency and number of UI events. An intake >4 L/day mandates consideration for diabetes insipidus, and small, frequent voids may indicate interstitial cystitis.

Urodynamic testing is often advocated for patients who have a history of mixed incontinence (i.e., both stress and urge symptoms). Using pressure catheters in the bladder and the vagina or rectum (as a surrogate for abdominal pressure), one can observe pressure abnormalities during filling/storage and voiding, and objectively document detrusor overactivity. Uroflowmetry measures the rate of urine flow when the patient is asked to spontaneously void and may provide useful information in patients with urinary hesitancy, incomplete emptying, or urinary retention. A simple cystometrogram involves placement of a urinary catheter to fill the bladder with sterile saline until the patient reaches capacity (normal: 300 to 700 mL). Detrusor contraction may be grossly observed, and a cough stress test is performed once the catheter is removed.

Imaging

Some clinicians advocate a voiding cystourethrogram in patients with UI and/or pelvic organ prolapse to assess for fistulas, to measure urethral hypermobility, and to grade the severity of cystoceles or bladder prolapse. Office cystoscopy may be performed in patients with new urgency and a frequency or worsening of UI complaints after pelvic surgery to assess for bladder stones, tumors, foreign bodies, fistulae, or urethral diverticula. If a urethral diverticulum is truly suspected, pelvic magnetic resonance imaging is the most sensitive imaging modality.

Treatment

The goals of treatment are to reduce symptoms and to improve the quality of life using nonsurgical and surgical therapies. Nonsurgical therapy may begin with lifestyle interventions such as stopping smoking and weight loss with moderate exercise. In morbidly obese patients, weight loss can reduce SUI—and to some extent—UUI (5).

Nonsurgical Therapies

The primary nonsurgical therapies include pelvic floor muscle training and bladder training, pharmacotherapy, and pessaries.

Pelvic Floor Muscle Training and Bladder Training. Pelvic floor muscle training (PFMT) uses exercises to gradually increase the strength of the pelvic floor muscles and may be augmented with vaginal weights, electrical stimulation, and formal biofeedback. Conscious squeezing of the levator ani muscles may be used before a cough or sneeze to prevent SUI, and "quick flicks" of the muscles may be used as a means of urge suppression along with distraction and relaxation for patients with UUI. Women with UI undergoing PFMT are 7 times more likely to be cured and 23 times more likely to show improvement than women not performing exercises (6). Besides PFMT, patients with UUI require more extensive "bladder training." Avoiding common bladder irritants (previously discussed) is a good first step. It is helpful to try scheduled voiding for women with urinary frequency by steadily increasing the time between voids. For example, start with hourly voids during waking hours and increase by 15 to 30 minutes per week until a 2- to 3-hour voiding interval is achieved. Bladder training and PFMT is best performed by a motivated patient with the assistance of a trained therapist who can guide and encourage the patient.

Pharmacotherapy. Pharmacotherapy predominantly is used for the treatment of UUI. Anticholinergic drugs such as oxybutynin and tolterodine are first-line agents that work by reducing detrusor contractions mediated by acetylcholine. These drugs effectively reduce the symptoms of urgency and improve the quality of life when compared with or combined with bladder training alone (7). Common side effects include dry mouth and constipation, which may limit the use of these drugs unless concomitant therapy for constipation is provided. Pharmacologic therapy for SUI is not as effective as surgical interventions, but some patients get a partial relief of symptoms with alpha-adrenergic agonists. The selective norepinephrine reuptake inhibitor, duloxetine, shows promise for the treatment of SUI, but is not yet approved by the Food and Drug Administration for this indication in the United States. Imipramine, a tricyclic antidepressant, may reduce detrusor contractility and increase outlet resistance, and can be used in conjunction with anticholinergics for UUI or SUI.

Pessaries. The primary devices used for the nonsurgical treatment of SUI include tampons or pessaries, which are intravaginal devices that support pelvic organs. After an appropriate fit is made to assure comfort and the relief of symptoms, patients are taught to remove the pessary regularly for cleaning and then place them back into the vaginal canal. Approximately half of women successfully fitted with a pessary will use it with improved symptoms for at least 1 to 2 years (8).

Surgical Therapies

A long history of more than 100 surgical procedures exists for the treatment of SUI. The gold standard surgeries include the Burch colposuspension and the fascial sling, both of which work to increase urethral support. The fascial sling has slightly higher cure rates than the Burch procedure at 2 years but results in more adverse events, including urinary tract infection, voiding dysfunction, and symptoms of overactive bladder (9). Newer minimally invasive midurethral slings have comparatively less recovery time than either of these other surgical procedures. One such sling, the tension-free vaginal tape appears to have similar long-term success rates as the Burch colposuspension. All surgical procedures for SUI carry risks of developing overactive bladder symptoms, voiding dysfunction, urinary retention, and urinary tract infection.

Surgical therapies are emerging for UUI patients who are refractory to more conservative management. Sacral neuromodulation involves the placement of a subcutaneous implant that provides electrical stimulation to sacral nerve roots to cause detrusor relaxation through an as-yet unknown mechanism; most patients may achieve at least a 50% improvement in symptoms with this therapy (10). Cystoscopic intravesical injection of botulinum toxin A may also result in temporary improvement in UUI.

Surgeries of last resort for UI include bladder augmentation or ileal conduit urinary diversion procedures. Urinary fistulae and urethral diverticula also require surgical repair.

EXTENDED IN-HOSPITAL MANAGEMENT

The newer midurethral slings (e.g., the tension-free vaginal tape) for SUI and sacral neuromodulation techniques for UUI are generally performed as outpatient surgery and do not require prolonged hospitalization. The Burch colposuspension and traditional pubovaginal fascial slings, on the other hand, may require a day or more of inpatient observation and several days of catheter drainage. It is important to monitor for signs of urinary outflow obstruction after any procedure that may result in urethral kinking, stenosis, or obstruction that causes bladder overdistention and sometimes overflow incontinence. Postoperative overdistention and urine leakage can also result from the prolonged effects of epidural anesthesia.

DISPOSITION

Discharge Goals

As for any gynecologic surgery, standard goals after UI surgery include having the patient ambulate, the return of gastrointestinal function, and achieving good pain control. In addition, an "active bladder test" is usually performed on the day of discharge by retrograde filling of the bladder with approximately 300 mL of sterile fluid and then removing the catheter to have the patient void. If the patient is able to void one half to two thirds of the volume instilled and does not feel bladder fullness, she is able to be discharged home without a catheter.

Outpatient Care

Postoperatively, if the patient is voiding normally, clinic follow-up is in approximately 1 month to check surgical incision sites. Patients who are discharged with indwelling catheters usually return within a week of surgery for an outpatient active bladder test. After SUI procedures, all patients should be observed for infection, voiding dysfunction, and de novo UUI.

 WHAT YOU NEED TO REMEMBER

- Stress and urge UI are the most common two types of UI, but it is important to evaluate for transient causes of incontinence ("DIAPPERS") and anatomic abnormalities such as vesicovaginal fistulae and urethral diverticula.
- Urinary incontinence evaluation requires a thorough medical, surgical, and obstetric history with a detailed pelvic exam to assess for abnormalities in neural function, anatomic abnormalities, and

urethral hypermobility. Urinalysis and documenting the PVR should be a part of the initial workup of UI.

- Stress urinary incontinence involves leakage with cough, sneeze, or exertion, and results from decreased anatomic support of the urethra. It may be managed with PFMT and medications that increase urethral sphincter closure pressure but often requires surgical therapy with either a Burch colposuspension or a sling procedure.

- Urge urinary incontinence is usually accompanied by urinary urgency, frequency, and nocturia. It is managed with a combination of bladder training, PFMT, and medications with surgical therapies for patients' refractory to standard management.

REFERENCES

1. Abrams P, Cardozo L, Fall M, et al. The standardization of terminology of lower urinary tract function: report from the Standardization Sub-committee of the International Continence Society. *Am J Obstet Gynecol.* 2002;187:116–126.
2. Nygaard IE, Heit M. Stress urinary incontinence. *Obstet Gynecol.* 2004;104:607–620.
3. Rogers RG. Urinary stress incontinence in women. *New Engl J Med.* 2008;358:1029.
   Rogers RG. Urinary stress incontinence in women. *New Engl J Med.* 2008;358(10):1029–1036.
4. Bent AE, Swift SE, Cundiff GW. *Ostergard's Urogynecology and Pelvic Floor Dysfunction.* 6th ed. Philadelphia: Lippincott Williams & Wilkins; 2008:65–77.
5. Subak LL, Whitcomb E, Shen H, et al. Weight loss: a novel and effective treatment for urinary incontinence. *J Urol.* 2005;174:190–195.
6. Hay-Smith EJ, Bo Berghmans LC, Hendricks HJ, et al. Pelvic floor muscle training for urinary incontinence in women. *Cochrane Database Syst Rev.* 2001;(1):CD001407.
7. Alhasso AA, McKinlay J, Patrick K, et al. Anticholinergic drugs versus non-drug active therapies for overactive bladder syndrome in adults. *Cochrane Database Syst Rev.* 2006;(4):CD003193.
8. Clemons JL, Aguilar VC, Sokol ER, et al. Patient characteristics that are associated with continued pessary use versus surgery after 1 year. *Am J Obstet Gyencol.* 2004;191:159–164.
9. Albo ME, Richter HE, Brubaker L, et al. Burch colposuspension versus fascial sling to reduce stress urinary incontinence. *N Engl J Med.* 2007;356:2143–2155.
10. Latini JM, Alipour M, Kreder KJ Jr. Efficacy of sacral neuromodulation for symptomatic treatment of refractory urinary urge incontinence. *Urology.* 2006;67:550–553.

Abnormal Pap Smear and Cervical Cancer

THE PATIENT ENCOUNTER

A 35-year-old woman (G6P2) presents to your office complaining of postcoital spotting. This problem has been going on for the last 6 months. She notes that she does not like going to the doctor and has not had a Pap smear since the birth of her last child 6 years ago.

OVERVIEW

Definition

The Pap smear is a screening test for early signs of cervical abnormalities. Cervical dysplasia is a loss in the uniformity and/or architectural orientation of individual epithelial cells. Cervical carcinoma may be a squamous cell carcinoma, arising from the lining epithelium, or adenocarcinoma, arising from glandular cells. The malignant cells have undergone molecular and cellular transformation, are able to grow independently, and are capable of local invasion with distant spread.

Pathophysiology

The human papillomavirus (HPV) is a nonenveloped papovaviridae virus. Presently, there are more than 100 genotypes of the HPV virus. There are approximately 40 known HPV types that infect the genital tract. Its circular, double-stranded DNA viral genome is composed of three parts. The late (L) region of the genome is for viral capsid expression. The early (E) region and the long regulatory protein region (LRR) insert to the host cell genome and controls transcription and replication of the viral genetic material. The E region has two important reading frames, E6 and E7, which play a very important role in the perpetual and uncontrolled growth of infected host cells that lead to malignancy.

CLINICAL PEARL

Cervical cancer is significantly associated with a persistent HPV infection.

In normal cells, there is homeostatic balance between two sets of genes: (i) protooncogenes versus tumor suppressor genes, and (ii) DNA repair versus apoptosis genes. The HPV alters the tumor suppressor retinoblastoma (*RB*) gene and the *p53* gene. In normal cells, the *RB* gene regulates cell cycles by inhibiting E2F, a family of transcription factors. The HPV E7 binds to the *RB* gene, producing disinhibition of transcription factors that lead to infinite cell-cycle progression. The *p53* gene controls cell cycle arrest and programmed cell death by stimulating the "growth arrest and DNA damage" gene and the apoptotic genes *p21* and *BAX*. Both HPV E6 and E7 bind to *p53* and *p21*, blocking apoptosis, and remove the restraints to cell proliferation.

As elaborate as the tumorigenesis it may seem, there are only approximately 12 high-risk HPV serotypes (e.g., 16, 18, and 31) that are associated with cancer. Most high-risk HPV infections clear within a few months and do not develop cancer.

Epidemiology

Worldwide, cervical cancer is the third most common cancer and it is the second most frequent cause of cancer death in women. In the United States, there is a significant decrease in incidence and mortality. In 2008, the incidence was estimated to be 11,150. The deaths were estimated at 3,850 (1).

The lifetime risk of for an individual to acquire HPV is at least 80%. Incidentally, cervical intraepithelial neoplasia (CIN) can occur within months of being exposed to the virus. Nevertheless, it takes on average between 8 and 12.6 years for a CIN 3 lesion to become invasive cancer (2). However, regression rates to normal cytology for CIN 1 and CIN 2 are 70% and 40%, respectively. (CIN lesions are further discussed in the section "Physical Examination.")

Etiology

The HPV is the central causative agent of cervical neoplasia and cancer. Other epidemiologic risk factors are early age at first sexual intercourse, multiple sexual partners, low socioeconomic status, and suppressed immunity (such as human immunodeficiency virus infection) (3).

ACUTE MANAGEMENT AND WORKUP

Diagnostic tests aid in the early detection of cervical dysplasia and the prevention of cervical cancer. The first encounter of a patient with cervical disease should focus on making a clear histologic diagnosis to assist with counseling and treatment planning.

The First 15 Minutes

In general, most patients with cervical dysplasia are asymptomatic. Rarely will patients present with postcoital bleeding or generalized pelvic pain.

Establishing a rapport with the patient and assessing for hemodynamic stability should be the goal of the first 15 minutes.

Initial Assessment

If vaginal bleeding is the primary complaint, the initial history is geared toward quantifying the amount and the extent of bleeding. Ask about the duration of bleeding, the subjective quantity of hemorrhage, any associated symptoms, and symptoms suggestive of hemodynamic instability.

Admission Criteria and Level of Care Criteria

A patient would only need to be admitted to the hospital if she had acute blood loss anemia with signs of systemic decompensation.

The First Few Hours

An assessment of risk and a complete physical exam are critical to the proper clinical staging of cervical cancer.

History

Most patients with CIN and early cervical cancer are asymptomatic. Symptomatic patients may present with vaginal bleeding, and some postcoital, watery, foul discharge. Tumors involving the pelvis may produce vague lower abdominal pain. If there is bladder involvement, your patient may complain of frank hematuria.

When taking the patient's history, it is important to elicit factors that increase the patient's risk for cervical neoplasia or cancer, such as smoking, risky sexual behavior, a history of sexually transmitted diseases, and immunosuppression.

Physical Examination

For CIN lesions, the cervix may be grossly normal. The colposcopic examination findings will be discussed in the section "The Pap Smear and The Bethesda System."

Cervical cancer infiltrates locally and spreads hematogenously. Supraclavicular, axillary, and inguinal nodes may be palpable. A careful speculum exam of the vagina may show a bleeding, ulcerating, or fungating cervical mass. A rectovaginal exam will allow you to examine the parametrial areas to assess for lateral spread of disease.

Labs and Tests to Consider

The key tests to consider when dealing with cervical dysplasia are the Pap smear, directed cervical biopsies, and endocervical curettage.

The Pap Smear and The Bethesda System

The Pap smear obtains endocervical cells with the use of a brush and ectocervical cells using a spatula. The collected sample is put on a glass slide, fixed with alcohol, and stained. Recently, a liquid-based system has been devised. The sample is placed in a liquid medium and is processed in the laboratory. This method slightly increases the sensitivity of the Pap smear. But more importantly, this system can facilitate HPV DNA testing to identify low-risk and high-risk serotypes.

The Bethesda System for reporting cervical cytology was developed to standardize the terminologies in the Pap smear report. According to the 2001 system, there were five key components: (i) specimen adequacy, (ii) general categorization, (ii) interpretation/results, (iv) automated review and ancillary testing, and (v) educational notes and suggestions (4). The 2006 Guidelines updated the indications for HPV testing and provided specific recommendations for three special populations of women: adolescents, pregnant patients, and postmenopausal women (5).

The interpretation categories adopted at the 2001 workshop remain unchanged after the 2006 workshop. Squamous epithelial cell abnormalities are broken up into two basic groups: atypical squamous cells and squamous intraepithelial lesions. The other subset of lesions is glandular in origin.

The equivocal groups of interpretations are lumped into the "atypical squamous cell" category. Atypical squamous cells of undetermined significance (ASC-US) and atypical squamous cell/cannot exclude high-grade squamous intraepithelial lesion (HSIL; ASC-H) are the least reproducible interpretations with a low prevalence of invasive cancer (0.5% to 2%) (5). The category is still used because moderate-to-severe dysplasia is found in 20% to 30% of these Pap smears (6).

The squamous cell lesions are reported using a two-tiered classification: low-grade squamous intraepithelial lesion (LSIL) and HSIL. The two abnormal squamous interpretations are very reproducible. In general, LSIL is indicative of a transient HPV infection whereas HSIL is associated with a persistent infection at higher risk of progression to invasive cancer.

Glandular abnormalities are classified as being endometrial, atypical endocervical, or glandular cells. The atypical glandular cell interpretation is associated with a higher incidence of severe dysplasia when compared with atypical squamous cell interpretations.

Colposcopy and Histologic Abnormalities

Abnormalities in Pap smear cytology should prompt you to further investigate the cervix in search of invasive cancer. Colposcopy is a test performed to obtain more information about the abnormal cells of the cervix. Colposcopy is performed in your office much like a Pap smear, except that you use a colposcope, which uses a binocular microscope, to carefully view the entire cervix. The most important area to visualize on the cervix is the transformation zone, which is the area between normal columnar epithelium and mature squamous epithelium. This zone of the cervix is where rapid cell turnover occurs and dysplasia commonly begins. Findings on colposcopy that warrant biopsy include cervical ulcerations, mosaic patterns, and vascular punctations.

The obtained cervical biopsies should be sent for pathologic evaluation for a histologic diagnosis. The diagnosis can range from normal to invasive cancer. Dysplasia is typically reported on a three-tiered scale: CIN 1 (mild dysplasia), CIN 2 (moderate dysplasia), and CIN 3 (severe dysplasia) (Fig. 27-1). The correlation between cervical cytology and biopsy histology help direct the future treatment plans.

Treatment

After you compare the results of your Pap smear and colposcopic biopsies, you are left with three basic follow-up options: (i) repeat cytology, (ii) HPV DNA testing, or (iii) a diagnostic excisional procedure.

Repeat cytology is an acceptable method of following patients with CIN 1 on biopsy with a Pap smear that was ASC-US, ASC-H, or LSIL. The cytology evaluation should be performed every 6 to 12 months until you have two negative results, after which you can switch the patient back to routine Pap screening. If your repeat cytology is ever abnormal, you would start the workup for an abnormal Pap smear again and perform colposcopy. In the special case of an adolescent woman (<21 years old) with CIN 1, you can basically watch one abnormal Pap screening and simply repeat the cytology evaluation in 12 months. If the first repeat Pap smear is <HSIL, you can wait and perform the second Pap smear 12 months later. If that Pap smear is negative, you can return to routine screening and should reserve colposcopy only for those with a persistently abnormal Pap smear.

The HPV DNA testing can be used to shorten the follow-up course of your patient with a cervical abnormality. For example, if your patient had CIN 1 on biopsy with a Pap smear that was ASC-US, ASC-H, or LSIL, you could simply perform an HPV DNA test in 12 months. If that test is negative, you can proceed with routine Pap screening. The HPV DNA testing can also be used for surveillance after a diagnostic excisional procedure. Excisional treatment includes performing a loop electrosurgical excision procedure (LEEP) or a cold knife cone. The LEEP is performed in the office using a local paracervical block. The cold knife conization is performed in the operating room using a scalpel directed toward the endocervix to core out a cone-shaped specimen. Both techniques produce a large specimen that is sent for pathologic evaluation. Each technique has an advantage and disadvantage when compared to the other. For example, the advantage of the LEEP is the ability to perform the procedure in the office without general anesthesia. On the other hand, the cold knife cone produces a biopsy free of cautery artifact at the margins (because you are performing the procedure with a scalpel). After the excision, acceptable follow-up approaches include two Pap smears at 6-month intervals or one HPV DNA test 6 to 12 months after treatment. Any positive finding should be further evaluated with colposcopy.

Descriptive Convention	Class I (normal)	Class II inflammation	Class III Mild dysplasia or Moderate dysplasia		Class IV severe dysplasia CIS	Class V suggestive of cancer or CIS
Class system	Class I (normal)	Class II inflammation	Mild dysplasia or Moderate dysplasia		Class IV severe dysplasia CIS	Class V suggestive of cancer or CIS
CIN system	Normal	Inflammatory	CIN I or CIN II		CIN III	Suggestive of cancer
Bethesda II system	Within normal limits	a. Without atypia b. With atypia or cellular changes associated with HPV	LSIL or HSIL		HSIL	Squamous cell cancer
Bethesda 2001	Negative for intraepithelial lesion or malignancy	ASC-US ASC-H	LSIL	HSIL		Squamous cell Carcinoma
Histology	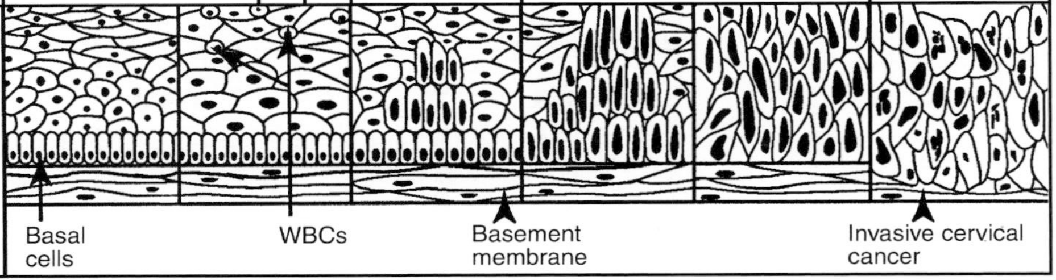 Basal cells	WBCs	LSIL	HSIL		Squamous cell Carcinoma

FIGURE 27-1: Comparison of Pap smear descriptive conventions.

EXTENDED IN-HOSPITAL MANAGEMENT

Precancerous cervical lesions are managed in the outpatient arena. In contrast, cervical cancer therapy is significantly more extensive and may require in-hospital care.

Staging for Cancer

The diagnosis of cervical cancer is established by biopsy. The clinical staging of cervical cancer involves palpation of the primary tumor and lymph nodes, colposcopy, excisional pathology, cystoscopy, hysteroscopy, proctoscopy, intravenous pyelogram, and plain radiographs of the lungs and bones. Please refer to Appendix 3 for the staging criteria of cervical cancer.

> ## CLINICAL PEARL
>
> *Unlike all other gynecologic cancers, cervical cancer is staged clinically as opposed to surgically.*

The Treatment of Cervical Cancer

The treatment of cervical cancer should be performed by an experienced gynecologic oncologist. Stage IA (IA1 and IA2) cervical cancer lesions are referred to as *microinvasive disease*. They carry a minor risk of lymph node involvement and generally respond excellently to treatment. In a young patient who wishes to preserve her fertility, a stage IA1 cervical cancer can be treated with a cervical conization alone. Once childbearing is no longer an issue, a simple hysterectomy is sufficient to treat this early stage of cervical cancer.

Patients with a lesion depth >3 mm but <5 mm are treated with a modified radical hysterectomy (which entails removal of the cervix, the proximal vagina, and paracervical and parametrial tissue) and a pelvic lymphadenectomy.

You can treat stage IB to IIA cervical cancer with either surgery (radical hysterectomy and pelvic lymphadenectomy) or primary radiotherapy. Surgery is usually done for younger patients who like to preserve their ovarian and sexual function.

Treatment of late-stage cancer (IIB or greater) is usually with external-beam and intracavitary (brachytherapy) radiation therapy. The addition of chemotherapy agents (such as the cisplatin-containing drugs) to radiotherapy improves the overall survival and disease-free survival rates.

DISPOSITION

Discharge Goals

After treatment with radiation or surgery, close surveillance is warranted for cervical cancer. Tumors are expected to shrink after 3 months of radiation. Eighty percent of recurrences after surgery are seen after 2 years. Posttreatment assessments should include a careful pelvic and rectal examination along with palpation of the supraclavicular, axillary, and inguinal lymph nodes. A cervical or vaginal cuff Pap smear is done every 3 months for 2 years and then every 6 months for 3 years.

Outpatient Care

The American College of Obstetricians and Gynecologists recommends that all women have their first Pap smear within 3 years of their first sexual intercourse or at age 21. Testing should be done annually until age 30. After 30 years of age, if there is no previous HSIL and the most recent tests have been normal, it may be performed every 2 to 3 years. For a patient who underwent a total hysterectomy (with the cervix surgically removed as well), as long as she has no history of HSIL or is not immunocompromised, testing is not recommended. Cytology sampling may be discontinued between the ages of 65 and 70.

Recently, a quadrivalent vaccine against the HPV has been approved by the Food and Drug Administration for women between the ages of 9 and 26. The four HPV genotypes covered are 6, 11, 16, and 18; HPV 6 and 11 account for approximately 90% of all cases of genital warts and HPV 16 and 18 are responsible for approximately 70% of cervical cancer cases. The vaccination is a three-part series is given at 0, 2, and 6 months. Testing for HPV is not recommended before vaccination (7).

CLINICAL PEARL

The HPV vaccine should be targeted at women between the ages of 11 and 13. The vaccine is most effective when given to women before the onset of sexual activity but is still beneficial in others.

WHAT YOU NEED TO REMEMBER

- The screening test of choice for cervical cancer is the Pap smear. It should be initiated when a patient turns 21 or within 3 years of her first sexual intercourse.
- The HPV is responsible for 99.7% of all cervical cancers.

- Risk factors for cervical cancer include smoking, immunosuppression, and having multiple sexual partners.
- Cervical cancer is staged clinically, not surgically.
- Colposcopy is an office procedure aimed at evaluating abnormal Pap smears. Colposcopy allows for directed biopsies of suspicious lesions.
- Periodic Pap smears may be discontinued between the ages of 65 and 70.

REFERENCES

1. American Cancer Society. Cervical cancer. Available at: http://www.cancer.org. Accessed December 1, 2008.
2. American College of Obstetricians and Gynecologists. ACOG practice bulletin number 99: management of abnormal cervical cytology and histology. *Obstet Gynecol.* 2008;112:1419–1444.
3. Katz VL, Lobo RA, Lentz GM, et al. *Comprehensive Gynecology.* 5th ed. Philadelphia: Mosby Elsevier, 2007;28:743–758; 29:759–780.
4. Solomon D, Schiffman M, Tarone R, for the ALTS Group. Comparison of three management strategies for patients with atypical squamous cells of undetermined significance: baseline results from a randomized trial. *J Natl Cancer Inst.* 2001;93:293–299.
5. Wright TC Jr, Massad LS, Dunton CJ, et al. 2006 consensus guidelines for the management of women with abnormal cervical cancer screening tests. 2006 American Society for Colposcopy and Cervical Pathology-sponsored Consensus Conference. *Am J Obstet Gynecol.* 2007;197:346–355.
6. Solomon D, Davey D, Kurman R, et al. The 2001 Bethesda System: terminology for reporting results of cervical cytology. *JAMA.* 2002;287:2114–119.
7. American College of Obstetrics and Gynecology. ACOG committee opinion number 344: Human papillomavirus vaccination. *Obstet Gynecol.* 2006;108:699–705.

SUGGESTED READINGS

American College of Obstetricians and Gynecologists. ACOG practice bulletin number 35: diagnosis and treatment of cervical carcinomas. *Obstet Gynecol.* 2002;99:855–867.
American College of Obstetricians and Gynecologists. ACOG practice bulletin number 45: cervical cytology screening. *Obstet Gynecol.* 2003;102:417–427.

Ovarian Cancer

A 56-year-old woman (G1P1) comes to your office complaining of mild abdominal pain. She tells you that she has been trying to exercise more but has to keep increasing her dress size. She notes that her appetite has been poor and what little she does eat fills her up pretty quickly. Something just does not make sense to her and she wanted to get checked out by you.

OVERVIEW

Definition

Ovarian cancer is overgrowth of abnormal ovarian cells. The ovary has three basic types of cells: (i) epithelial cells, which cover the ovary; (ii) stromal cells, which are connective tissue where estrogen and progesterone are made; and (iii) germ cells, which are cells that make eggs (Table 28-1). Nearly 85% of all ovarian cancers are epithelial in origin.

Pathophysiology

The exact etiology of ovarian cancer has not been identified. Ovulation has been theorized to increase the risk of ovarian cancer because we do know that oral contraceptive pills and pregnancy can reduce the risk of ovarian cancer. A lot of research has been done to describe the two most common genetic mutations that can increase a woman's risk of getting breast and ovarian cancer. Radiation and chemical exposures that cause DNA mutations have not been clearly linked to ovarian cancer.

CLINICAL PEARL

Women with a BRCA1 gene mutation have a 30% to 70% lifetime risk of developing ovarian cancer; for women with the BRCA2 gene, the lifetime risk is between 10% and 30%.

TABLE 28-1
Types of Ovarian Tumors

Tissue Type	Most Common Tumor
Epithelial	Serous carcinomas
	Mucinous carcinomas
	Endometrioid carcinomas
	Clear cell carcinomas
Stromal	Granulose cell tumors
	Granulose-theca tumors
	Sertoli-Leydig cell tumors
Germ cell	Dysgerminomas
	Endodermal sinus tumors
	Choriocarcinomas

Epidemiology

According to the American Cancer Society, ovarian cancer accounts for approximately 3% of all cancers in women, with over 21,500 new cases diagnosed in 2008. Ovarian cancer is the eighth most commonly occurring cancer among women and the fifth leading cause of cancer-related death in women. Ovarian cancer afflicts women beyond the fifth decade of life.

Etiology

Although the exact cause of ovarian cancer has not been isolated, there are a number of risk factors that increase the chances of your patient developing ovarian cancer. The three most widely recognized unmodifiable risk factors are age, a personal history of breast cancer, and a family history of breast, ovary, or colorectal cancer. A number of modifiable risk factors have been identified with which you can help your patient. Obesity not only increases your patient's risk of developing ovarian cancer but it also increases her risk of mortality. Having children, using oral contraceptive pills, and breast-feeding lower a woman's risk of ovarian cancer. Finally, the use of talcum powder on or near the genital area has been suggested to increase the risk of ovarian cancer.

ACUTE MANAGEMENT AND WORKUP

The issue that most acutely plagues patients with ovarian cancer is a small bowel obstruction (SBO). Anyone complaining of nausea, vomiting, and an inability to tolerate oral intake in the face of a pelvic mass should raise your suspicions and lower your threshold for in-hospital admission.

The First 15 Minutes

When a patient presents with severe nausea and vomiting from a partial SBO, the initial assessment made from your patient's general appearance is usually correct. If your patient is dehydrated and suffers from advanced cancer, she will appear gaunt and fatigued.

Initial Assessment

A patient with severe dehydration will complain of feeling light-headed, weak, and even confused. Tachycardia will be present upon initial vital signs. Be sure to check your patient's temperature to exclude an infectious etiology.

Admission Criteria and Level of Care Criteria

If your patient has failed outpatient attempts at rehydration or clearly cannot tolerate sips of liquids, she should be admitted for intravenous hydration and electrolyte repletion. The level of acuity could change if your initial imaging studies suggest a complete bowel obstruction or rupture of a viscous organ.

The First Few Hours

After you have stabilized your patient's acute issue, the next part of your assessment is aimed at trying to establish the cause of her SBO. Not all pelvic masses are cancer, and a thorough history and physical exam can help you stratify the patient's risk for cancer.

History

After your patient has been admitted and stabilized, you should spend some time reviewing the patient's symptom history in conjunction with as assessment of her risk factors for ovarian cancer. If the disease has spread beyond the ovaries and pelvis, you patient may have persistent complaints of bloating, fatigue, abdominal pain, or difficulty with eating. If your index of suspicion is high for ovarian cancer, it is advisable to discuss the case with a gynecologic oncologist to help coordinate care efforts and minimize any unnecessary tests.

Physical Examination

Because ovarian cancer is a surgically staged disease, a complete physical exam is necessary to not only predict the extent of disease but also to help optimize your patient's conditions prior to surgery. Most women with ovarian cancer will be older and will have multiple comorbidities. A careful cardiopulmonary exam is essential to minimize operative risks.

Labs and Tests to Consider

In general, the only laboratory tests necessary are those indicated by your patient's medical comorbidities. A complete blood count, basic metabolic panel, and blood type/screen are the most common laboratory tests obtained. Depending on the extent of disease, it would not be unreasonable to have the blood bank hold a couple of units of cross-matched blood products in the event of a difficult surgery.

A CA-125 level, although not predictive, is usually obtained preoperatively to help follow your patient's response to chemotherapy.

> **CLINICAL PEARL**
>
> *A CA-125 is not a good screening test for ovarian cancer. Many other processes can result in a false-positive finding, such as endometriosis, pelvic inflammatory disease, pregnancy, and even fibroids.*

Imaging

Preoperative imaging studies will not help determine a patient's cancer stage. The value of imaging studies is to assess the extent of disease and organs possibly involved. The two most common tests obtained are pelvic ultrasound and computed tomography (CT) scan. Ultrasound should provide information on elements such as the complexity and size of the lesion, bilateralism, and the presence of extraovarian disease.

The CT scan can better identify suspected lymph nodes and organs outside the pelvis that may be involved in the disease process. In the face of an uncertain diagnosis, a CT-guided biopsy is helpful.

Treatment

Ovarian cancer is a surgically staged gynecologic cancer. The type of treatment depends on a patient's surgical type and stage. In general, the main categories of therapy are surgery, chemotherapy, and radiation therapy.

Surgical Therapy

The main goal of surgical intervention is confirming the patient's stage and minimizing the burden of disease (otherwise known as debulking). The lymphatic spread of ovarian cancer helps dictate where proper sampling should happen (Fig. 28-1). To properly stage ovarian cancer, your patient needs to have her uterus, both ovaries, both fallopian tubes, the omentum, peritoneal washings, diaphragmatic and multiple peritoneal biopsies, and complete pelvic and para-aortic lymphadenectomy (Appendix 3).

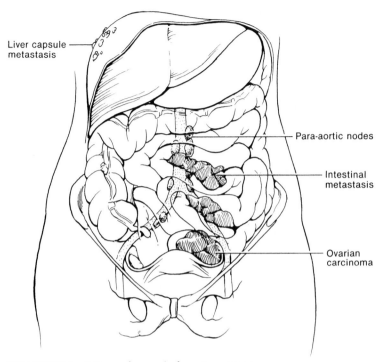

Liver capsule metastasis

Para-aortic nodes

Intestinal metastasis

Ovarian carcinoma

FIGURE 28-1: Pattern of spread of ovarian cancer.

The purpose of the debulking procedure is to maximally reduce the patient's tumor burden. Gynecologic oncologists strive to leave behind no tumor larger than 1 cm. In advanced cases of ovarian cancer, optimal debulking will require procedures such as a spleenectomy and even a bowel resection.

Chemotherapy

Systemic chemotherapy helps treat the microscopic disease and lengthen the disease-free interval. The medications most commonly used in ovarian cancer are paclitaxel and carboplatin. These drugs are administered for six cycles in 3- to 4-week intervals. The routes of delivery include intravenously and now intraperitoneally.

Radiation Therapy

With the discovery of effective chemotherapy, radiation therapy is now rarely used. The situations in which radiation therapy may still have a role are localized recurrences or if an ovarian cyst is ruptured at the time of surgery in an attempt to kill all of the cancer cells.

EXTENDED IN-HOSPITAL MANAGEMENT

After your patient has undergone a surgical staging and/or a debulking procedure, the recovery follows typical postoperative courses. If she had a lot of ascites or gastrointestinal (GI) involvement, she may have some electrolyte abnormalities postoperatively that will require attention.

DISPOSITION

Discharge Goals

The most common postoperative parameters used to determine when a patient can be discharged are return of GI function and pain control. Patients who have undergone a debulking procedure may have slow to return GI function, so be patient with their diet advancement and clearly confirm that they can stay hydrated at home. Unfortunately, pain medicine can complicate proper functioning of the GI tract so a fine balance has to be met. Prior to discharge from the hospital, a clear plan for outpatient treatment (chemotherapy) should be outlined.

Outpatient Care

A majority of ovarian cancers are found in the later stages of disease. Outpatient care for all women should incorporate strategies aimed at early detection of disease. Women should continue having annual pelvic exams regardless of the need for a Pap smear. No effective screening tests exist for ovarian cancer. Transvaginal ultrasounds can help characterize a mass felt on pelvic exam but its ability to distinguish cancer from benign conditions is limited. A serum CA-125 evaluation is only slightly helpful in women at very high risk for developing cancer. There are a number of entities that cause a falsely elevated CA-125 level, such as endometriosis, pelvic inflammatory disease, adenomyosis, and even pregnancy. In patients with a history of ovarian cancer, close attention to your patient's symptoms will help catch early recurrences. Patients with ovarian cancer will commonly have complaints such as abdominal swelling, bloating, pelvic pressure, difficulty eating, early satiety, or urge urinary symptoms.

WHAT YOU NEED TO REMEMBER

- CA-125 is not an effective screening test for ovarian cancer; it is usually obtained preoperatively to help follow your patient's response to chemotherapy.
- An annual pelvic exam is recommended for preventative health care.

- Epithelial ovarian cancers are the most common, representing approximately 85% of ovarian cancers.
- Symptoms that should raise your suspicion of ovarian cancer include persistent abdominal bloating, abdominal swelling, early satiety, and pelvic pressure.
- A gynecologic oncologist should be involved early in the care of a patient with suspected ovarian cancer to appropriately perform surgical debulking and staging.
- Ovarian cancer is the leading cause of death from a gynecologic cancer.

SUGGESTED READINGS

American College of Obstetricians and Gynecologists. ACOG committee opinion number 280: the role of the generalist obstetrician–gynecologist in the early detection of ovarian cancer. *Obstet Gynecol.* 2002;100:1413–1416.

American College of Obstetricians and Gynecologists. ACOG committee opinion number 396: intraperitoneal chemotherapy for ovarian cancer. *Obstet Gynecol.* 2008;111:249–251.

American Cancer Society. Ovarian cancer. Available at: http://www.cancer.org. Accessed November 19, 2008.

Coleman R, Gershenson D. Neoplastic diseases of the ovary: screening, benign and malignant epithelial and germ cell neoplasms, sex-cord stromal tumors. In: Katz VL, Lentz GM, Lobo RA, et al., eds. *Comprehensive Gynecology.* 5th ed. Philadelphia: Mosby Elsevier; 2007:839–883.

Endometrial Cancer

THE PATIENT ENCOUNTER

A 51-year-old woman (G1P1) presents to your clinic with a complaint of vaginal bleeding shortly after menopause. She notes the onset of vaginal spotting with occasional frank bleeding a month before her visit. She denies all constitutional symptoms, including night sweats, weight loss, and increased abdominal girth.

OVERVIEW

Definition

Postmenopausal bleeding is bleeding that occurs after a full 12 months of amenorrhea (i.e., menopause). Postmenopausal bleeding and abnormal bleeding in premenopausal and perimenopausal women are the most common presenting symptoms of endometrial cancer and should always prompt a full investigation of its cause, including, but not limited to, an endometrial biopsy.

Endometrial cancer refers to several types of malignancy that are described in greater detail within this chapter. The most common type is endometrioid adenocarcinoma.

Pathophysiology

Most endometrial cancers arise from epithelial cells that line the endometrium. The most common endometrioid type involves cancer cells growing in patterns reminiscent of normal endometrium. By contrast, the more aggressive yet fortunately less common papillary serous and clear cell types of endometrial carcinomas (<15% of all endometrial cancers) arise from different cellular types. Papillary serious endometrial carcinoma may develop from endometrial intraepithelial carcinoma, a lesion related to the malignant transformation of surface epithelium, such as a polyp, in an area of endometrial atrophy. Clear cell cancers, in turn, are characterized by tubulocystic, papillary, or solid patterns and psammoma bodies.

Epidemiology

Endometrial carcinoma is the most common gynecologic malignancy in the United States. Fortunately, most cases are diagnosed at an early stage as they present with postmenopausal bleeding, and surgery alone may be adequate for cure. Thus, endometrial carcinoma is only the third most common cause of gynecologic cancer death, falling behind ovarian and cervical cancer (1). Survival rates are estimated at 96% for localized disease, 67% for regional disease, and 23% for metastatic disease. Incidence rates of uterine corpus cancer are higher in whites than in other racial groups. However, mortality is almost two times higher in African Americans than in whites, perhaps because of a higher incidence of aggressive cancer subtypes (type II) or because of poor access to care and specialty surgeons (2).

Etiology

Two forms of endometrial carcinoma exist. Type I endometrial carcinoma is estrogen-dependent and presents in premenopausal and perimenopausal women with a history of unopposed estrogen. Histologically, it is a low-grade endometrioid tumor and is associated with atypical endometrial hyperplasia. Risk factors for type I include obesity, nulliparity, endogenous or exogenous estrogen excess, diabetes mellitus, and hypertension.

Type II endometrial carcinoma is not estrogen-dependent. It is more common in older, postmenopausal women, and African Americans. Type II endometrial cancers are high-grade endometrioid or cell types that carry a poor prognosis, including papillary serous and clear cell carcinomas. Type II endometrial carcinoma carries a much dimmer prognosis than type I.

Endometrial stromal sarcomas are endometrial cancers that originate in the nonglandular connective tissue of the endometrium. Sarcomas are more aggressive than endometrioid tumors. They occur primarily in women between 40 and 60 years of age and account for fewer than 4% of uterine malignancies. Uterine carcinosarcoma, previously termed *malignant mixed mullerian tumor*, is a rare and extremely aggressive uterine cancer that contains cancerous cells with both a glandular and a sarcomatous appearance.

ACUTE MANAGEMENT AND WORKUP

Although the majority of women with endometrial cancer will present with abnormal or postmenopausal bleeding, very few will have bleeding significant enough to prompt an acute workup.

The First 15 Minutes

As the diagnosis is tissue-based, a physician's primary responsibility in the face of a possible cancer diagnosis is to use the appropriate diagnostic tool to achieve the most accurate pathology and staging of disease, thereby prompting the correct treatment course, whether surgery, chemotherapy, or radiation (see the sections "Key Diagnostic Labs and Tests" and "Prognosis").

Initial Assessment

It is important to remember that the amount of bleeding does not correlate with the risk of cancer. Postmenopausal women with scant vaginal bleeding can be at high risk for cancer, depending on the risk factors present. If a patient presented with hypovolemic shock secondary to acute blood loss anemia, the initial assessment would focus first on achieving hemodynamic stability.

Admission Criteria and Level of Care Criteria

If you encounter the rare circumstance in which a patient is bleeding heavily and has signs of hypovolemic shock, you should admit this patient to the hospital for stabilization and a possible blood transfusion. Once the patient is stable, proceed to making a determination of the underlying cause of the bleeding. Other indications for admitting a patient with endometrial cancer would be severe pain unresponsive to outpatient therapy.

The First Few Hours

A thorough history and physical exam will allow the physician an opportunity to make the correct diagnosis and ensure a timely referral to a gynecologic oncologist.

History

Be sure to elicit from your patients any risk factors that might predispose them to endometrial cancer, including a family or personal history of ovarian, breast, colon, or endometrial cancer; tamoxifen use; chronic anovulation; obesity; estrogen therapy; prior endometrial hyperplasia; and diabetes mellitus. Risk factors can also be evaluated with a thought toward whether a patient is more likely to have type I or type II endometrial cancer.

You should also remember to ask about other constitutional symptoms associated with cancer, such as weight loss, decreased appetite, increased satiety, increased abdominal girth, and night sweats.

Physical Examination

You should always perform a full pelvic exam. Assess the size and position of the uterus, and whether any adnexal mass is palpable. Determine the extent of current bleeding and whether acute intervention is needed. Perform a complete breast exam and record the presence of palpable masses, noting mobility, quality, and location. Examine the patient's pulmonary and cardiovascular status. Determine if the patient is currently hemodynamically stable.

Labs and Tests to Consider

Because many of these patients require surgery, you should optimize any chronic medical conditions to minimize the risks associated with surgery. The main laboratory evaluations and tests you order will assist you during the preoperative workup.

Key Diagnostic Labs and Tests

Key diagnostic laboratory evaluations and tests include a comprehensive preoperative workup and endometrial sampling.

Preoperative Workup. In the event that a patient's biopsy is consistent with endometrial cancer, she will be referred to a gynecologic oncologist for surgical staging. A preoperative workup should include, as a baseline, a complete blood count, and basic serum chemistries. Given the risk of blood loss in a staging surgery, a baseline measure of hematocrit and creatinine levels is of greatest importance. A pregnancy test should be performed initially in all premenopausal and perimenopausal women, and should be repeated on the day of surgery. An electrocardiogram and a chest radiograph should be performed to screen for previously undetected cardiac or pulmonary disorders. If the patient is known to have underlying cardiac, pulmonary, or systemic disease, she should be referred to an internist for a full evaluation of her ability to tolerate major staging surgery and possible adjuvant chemotherapy and/or radiation.

A serum CA-125 level should be obtained in all women with endometrial cancer. Although an elevated CA-125 level may help you predict how much the disease has spread beyond the uterus, the main value of this laboratory test is to help you evaluate the patient's response to treatment.

Endometrial Sampling. Because endometrial cancer is a histologic diagnosis, tissue must be obtained as soon as possible. The most cost-effective method is a blind endometrial biopsy (EMB) that is performed in the office setting using a Pipelle sampling device. This procedure is well tolerated and has a low complication rate with a high sensitivity. Benign endometrial histology includes pathology findings of atrophy, proliferative endometrium (estrogen effect), secretory endometrium (progestin effect), disordered or dissynchronous endometrium, and endometritis.

If <50% of the endometrium is affected, a malignancy can be missed by an EMB. If an EMB fails to provide a diagnosis yet bleeding persists and the clinical suspicion is high, or if an EMB is not possible because of cervical stenosis or another barrier to sampling, an operative dilation and curettage may be performed to obtain tissue. If a patient is scheduled for a dilation and curettage, she should also be asked to consent to hysteroscopy as this study can aid in the detection of focal lesions of the endometrial lining that may otherwise be missed.

> ## CLINICAL PEARL
>
> *A thin endometrial stripe (<4 mm in postmenopausal women) is consistent with atrophy as a cause of minimal vaginal bleeding and is reassuring evidence against an underlying endometrial cancer.*

Imaging

If the EMB provides an inadequate sample and bleeding does not persist, a transvaginal sonogram may be performed.

Treatment

Surgical staging is the primary therapy for endometrial cancer (Appendix 3). Staging includes hysterectomy, bilateral salpingo-oophorectomy (BSO), cytologic exam of peritoneal fluid, biopsy of suspicious intraperitoneal or retroperitoneal lesions, and retroperitoneal lymph node sampling. The decision to perform a complete pelvic lymphadenectomy and an extended para-aortic node dissection rather than selective nodal sampling is a point of debate. If the risk of nodal metastasis is low, as with stage IA or IB cancer, and gross inspection and nodal palpation reveal nothing of concern, some experts advocate surgical staging limited to a total hysterectomy and bilateral salpingo-oophorectomy, omitting lymphadenectomy.

Bilateral salpingo-oophorectomy is performed to exclude adnexal micrometastases or synchronous tumors, and to remove the ovaries as a source of estrogen. Synchronous primary cancers of the endometrium and the ovary are found in up to 10% of women with ovarian cancer and in up to 5% of women with endometrial cancer.

Prognosis

The prognosis is determined by the disease stage and the histologic type (2). Certain pathologic findings are associated with an increased risk of extrauterine disease and recurrence after the initial therapy:

- Serous, clear cell, or high-grade endometrioid histology
- Myometrial invasion >50%
- Tumor extension beyond the uterine fundus
- Involvement of the lymphovascular space
- A larger tumor (>2 cm diameter; this is a controversial finding)

> ### CLINICAL PEARL
>
> *Because most women with endometrial cancer present with abnormal uterine bleeding, the disease is typically caught at an early stage and the prognosis (as compared with other gynecologic cancers) is optimistic.*

EXTENDED IN-HOSPITAL MANAGEMENT

Only those women who are hemodynamically unstable will require long-term in-hospital management. All other patients may be discharged home to await pathology results and surgical planning as appropriate.

If a previously unstable patient is stabilized after excessive bleeding and is admitted, she must be monitored for stabilization of her hematocrit level, the resolution of an acute bleeding episode, and the development of thrombotic complications from estrogen therapy (if used), especially pulmonary embolism. Prophylactic measures should be undertaken; compression devices are usually adequate.

The discussion of postoperative and postchemotherapy complications and their management is beyond the scope of this chapter.

DISPOSITION

Discharge Goals

Postsurgical care in the setting of endometrial cancer should maintain end points similar to any surgical procedure. Once gastrointestinal function and the ability to perform basic activities of daily living have been demonstrated, the patient may be allowed to recover in an outpatient setting. Frequently, patients with endometrial cancer are older and have other medical comorbidities that require optimization prior to discharge.

Outpatient Care

The risk of recurrence is greatest within the first 3 years of diagnosis. Clinical follow-up should include an assessment of symptoms associated with recurrence:

- Vaginal bleeding
- Abdominal or pelvic pain
- Persistent cough (up to 60% of recurrences occur in distant locations, including the upper abdomen and the lungs)
- Unexplained weight loss

Follow-up should include a physical exam every 3 to 6 months for 2 years and then annually. Vaginal cytology studies should be performed every

6 months for 2 years and then annually. Isolated vaginal vault recurrences are often curable. If the patient's initial CA-125 level was elevated, this test should be repeated during a follow-up visit.

WHAT YOU NEED TO REMEMBER

- Endometrial cancer is the most common gynecologic malignancy; however, it is curable. It is third in mortality behind ovarian and cervical cancer.
- Endometrial cancer is a surgically staged disease. Stage is the most important prognostic factor in endometrial cancer.
- The treatment for patients with a low and an intermediate risk (less than stage II cancer) is usually surgery alone. There is a possible role for radiation therapy in patients with an intermediate risk. Chemotherapy is an appropriate option for women with a high risk of recurrence.

REFERENCES

1. American Cancer Society. Available at: http://www.cancer.org/docroot/CRI/CRI_2_3x.asp? dt =11. Accessed November 23, 2008.
2. Sorosky JI. Endometrial cancer. *Obstet Gynecol.* 2008;111:436–447.

SUGGESTED READINGS

American College of Obstetricians and Gynecologists. ACOG practice bulletin number 65: management of endometrial cancer. *Obstet Gynecol.* 2005;106:413–425.
Schorge J, Schaffer J, Halvorson L, et al. Endometrial cancer. In: *Williams Gynecology.* New York: Mc-Graw Hill; 2008:687–706.

Gestational Trophoblastic Disease

THE PATIENT ENCOUNTER

A healthy 33-year-old woman (G4P3003) at 15 to 16 weeks of gestation by last menstrual period presents to the emergency department with vaginal bleeding and several episodes of nonbilious emesis for 1 week. She says her pregnancy has been uncomplicated thus far, but her private doctor has not been able to hear the fetal heart tones in the office.

OVERVIEW

Definition

Gestational trophoblastic disease (GTD) is a spectrum of disorders of the placenta that is derived from syncytiotrophoblasts and cytotrophoblastic cells. Gestational trophoblastic disease encompasses the conditions known as complete and partial hydatidiform moles, invasive moles, gestational choriocarcinoma, and placental site trophoblastic tumors. The latter three conditions and postmolar GTD are commonly referred to as *gestational trophoblastic neoplasia* or *malignant gestational trophoblastic disease*. This chapter will focus on the most common type of GTD, the hydatidiform mole.

The hydatidiform mole can persist as postmolar GTD, can invade the myometrium in the case of invasive moles, and can lead to metastases in the case of choriocarcinomas. A rare but histologically distinct variant of gestational trophoblastic neoplasia is a placental site trophoblastic tumor that is notoriously insensitive to chemotherapy. Gestational trophoblastic neoplasia usually follows some form of an antecedent pregnancy, commonly the hydatidiform mole, but can also follow normal term pregnancies, spontaneous abortions, or ectopic pregnancies. Postmolar GTD, invasive moles, choriocarcinoma, and placental site trophoblastic tumors are all types of malignant GTD or gestational trophoblastic neoplasia.

Pathophysiology

The typical chromosomal pattern for complete moles that have undergone androgenesis is 46 XX. If dispermic fertilization takes place, two sperm fertilize the empty ovum, which can result in 46, XY or 46, XX karyotype and accounts for approximately 5% of complete moles (1,2). Clinically, the serum beta-human chorionic gonadotropin (β-hCG) level is extremely elevated. Histologically, the complete mole typically displays diffuse hydropic degeneration and swelling of the chorionic villi, diffuse proliferation of the trophoblastic epithelium, and an absence of fetal cells. Complete moles have up to a 20% chance of progressing to gestational trophoblastic neoplasia.

Partial moles generally have a triploid chromosomal pattern of 69 XXX. However, 69 XXY does exist and results from dispermic fertilization of a haploid ovum. Although the majority of complete moles are diploid and most partial moles are triploid, other chromosomal patterns have been described. The serum β-hCG level for partial moles is generally much lower than complete moles and can be nearly normal or slightly elevated. Histologically, the villous edema and trophoblastic proliferation tends to be more focal in the partial mole than the complete mole, and fetal cells are usually present in the partial mole. Partial moles have a much lower likelihood, 2.5% to 7.5%, of progressing to GTD when compared with the complete moles (1,2). Table 30-1 provides the key features of complete and partial molar pregnancies.

TABLE 30-1
Key Features of Complete and Partial Molar Pregnancies

Characteristic	Complete Moles	Partial Moles
Karyotype	46, XX or 46, XY	69, XXX or 69, XXY
Fetal cells	Absent	Present
Chorionic villi	Diffusely hydropic	Focal, partial edema
Physical exam (fundal height)	50% are greater than dates	Small or appropriate for dates
Serum β-hCG	Extremely elevated	Normal or slightly elevated
Medical complications	Common	Rare
Postmolar GTN	6.8%–20%	2.5%–7.5%

β-hCG, beta-human chorionic gonadotropin; GTN, gestational trophoblastic neoplasia.

CLINICAL PEARL

Complete moles have a 20% chance of progressing to gestational trophoblastic neoplasia as compared with partial moles, which only carry a 2.5% to 7% risk. Therefore, patients with a complete molar pregnancy should be monitored closely for 6 to 12 months looking for GTD.

Epidemiology

In the United States, 1 in 600 elective abortions have subsequent pathologic diagnosis of a hydatidiform mole and, overall in the United States, 1 in 1,500 pregnancies are hydatidiform moles (3). The incidence has been reported to be higher in some Asian countries, such as Japan, where the incidence is reported to be 2 in 1,000 (1,2). Several risk factors exist that can increase the baseline risk of a hydatidiform mole, including age younger than 15 and older than 40, a history of a previous mole, protein malnourishment, and low socioeconomic status (1,2).

Etiology

Complete moles are usually formed by androgenesis but can form from dispermic fertilization. Androgenesis occurs when the ovum is fertilized by a haploid sperm that then duplicates its own chromosomes after meiosis. This phenomenon results in chromosomes derived only from paternal origin. The chromosomes of the ovum are either absent or inactivated. In contrast to the complete moles, partial moles are derived from both maternal and paternal sets of chromosomes.

ACUTE MANAGEMENT AND WORKUP

Establishing hemodynamic stability and the management of heavy vaginal bleeding are the two most important steps in the acute inpatient management of a patient with GTD.

The First 15 Minutes

The first step is to get a thorough but focused history.

Initial Assessment

Although vaginal bleeding is common to hydatidiform moles, it is a common and serious complaint of pregnancy. Thus, it is important to rule out other causes of vaginal bleeding during pregnancy, such as ectopic pregnancy and spontaneous abortion. The passage of any blood clots or tissue from the vagina that resembles grapes would raise your suspicion for a molar gestation.

Quantify the amount of blood loss that has occurred and over what period of time by asking the patient how many sanitary napkins she used and how often she is changing soiled sanitary napkins.

Admission Criteria and Level of Care Criteria

If your patient is symptomatic from acute blood loss anemia, admission for a blood transfusion and fluid resuscitation is mandatory. Measures to stop the bleeding will be discussed in the "Treatment" section.

The First Few Hours

After admission, the primary focus of the first few hours should be delineating the cause of vaginal bleeding and gathering the resources to initiate therapy.

History

A focused history in search of common medical complications related to hydatidiform moles will expedite this process. Palpitations may alert you to monitor for thyrotoxicosis. Ask the patient if she is having any symptoms of severe pre-eclampsia, such as a headache, vision changes, or right upper quadrant/epigastric pain.

Physical Examination

On physical examination, the first thing to notice is the patient's vital signs. Your patient may be tachycardic from acute blood loss anemia or volume depletion from vomiting, or she may have thyrotoxicosis, which can be a medical complication of complete hydatidiform moles. Do a focused physical exam, including a sterile speculum exam to check for the amount of blood in the vaginal vault and whether or not the cervical os is open, indicating an incomplete or an inevitable abortion. Assess the fundal height of the uterus. Attempt to get fetal heart tones on exam via Doppler study.

Labs and Tests to Consider

Laboratory data will be the next important piece of information in the initial workup of this patient. All pregnant women with vaginal bleeding should have a serum quantitative β-hCG test and blood group status checked on initial presentation. The β-hCG level for a molar pregnancy will typically be much higher than expected for gestational age. The peak value for β-hCG in normal, singleton pregnancies occurs at 10 to 14 weeks and rarely exceeds 100,000 mIU/mL. Useful preoperative data include a baseline complete blood count to screen for anemia, coagulation studies, thyroid function tests to screen for thyrotoxicosis, liver function testing, a baseline creatinine measure, and a chest radiograph to evaluate for metastatic disease. Serum electrolyte testing should also be obtained to screen for hyperemesis gravidarum, especially if severe nausea and vomiting are present.

Imaging

The next vital diagnostic tool is a pelvic ultrasound. The classic characteristics of a complete mole on ultrasound are a "snowstorm" appearance and diffuse, mixed inhomogeneous echoes that depict the hydropic changes in the placental tissue. Incomplete or partial moles can have fetal parts and even a fully developed fetus that accompanies the mole, so expert interpretation of the sonographic pictures is advised to confirm the diagnosis. During the sonogram, the ovaries should be evaluated as well because theca-lutein cysts can be seen in molar gestations, especially in complete moles. Theca-lutein cysts are thought to form from the high level of β-hCG that stimulates ovarian cells. These cysts can sometimes undergo torsion, infarct, and bleed, but they generally regress after evacuation of the molar gestation.

Treatment

Hydatidiform moles are best managed surgically. If a woman has completed her childbearing, then hysterectomy is recommended, otherwise a dilation and curettage is the standard initial treatment for molar pregnancies. However, prior to the operating room procedure, you should anticipate medical complications, especially in molar pregnancies ≥14 to 16 weeks (3). The goal of preoperative testing is to anticipate and stabilize as many clinical problems as possible prior to the invasive procedure. If severe anemia exists and the hematocrit level is ≤25%, you should consider preoperative blood transfusion because the surgical management of hydatidiform moles is known to result in significant blood loss. Despite the results of the hemoglobin or hematocrit testing, a type and crossmatch should be performed on all patients in the anticipation of a necessary blood transfusion. Two large-bore peripheral intravenous lines should also be established prior to the procedure.

During the evacuation of the hydatidiform mole via dilation and curettage, there are several helpful clinical pearls that can minimize operative time and complications. First, an abdominal ultrasound should be available during the procedure; it should be used to guide the evacuation in real time to ensure complete evacuation and to minimize the risk of uterine perforation. Next, one should choose the largest diameter suction curette to perform the procedure. Also, once the curettage begins, the surgeon should not take the curette out of the uterus while the suction canisters fill with molar tissue because this usually results in profuse bleeding and poor visualization. Instead, an assistant should quickly change each canister for the surgeon as it fills. Finally, it is important to communicate with the anesthesiologist and ask for the intravenous Pitocin to be initiated as soon as the procedure begins in order to allow the uterus to contract down and expel the tissue.

Although severe blood loss, high-output cardiac failure from thyroid storm or anemia, pulmonary embolism, and amniotic fluid embolism are some causes for cardiopulmonary complications during the procedure, one should also be aware that trophoblastic tissue has been documented to escape into the venous circulation, causing pulmonary embolism, massive pulmonary edema, and even metastatic disease in some case reports. These embolic complications are more common in larger hydatidiform moles (those greater in size than 14 to 16 weeks). At the culmination of a successful procedure, the uterus is generally much smaller than the preoperative exam and hemostasis is achieved.

EXTENDED IN-HOSPITAL MANAGEMENT

Postoperative care includes observing the trend in the hemoglobin and hematocrit levels to assess for further transfusion needs, and continuing the intravenous Pitocin in the initial hour after the procedure. All Rh-negative patients should receive RhoGAM because there is always the possibility of a partial mole being diagnosed from the final pathology report. Adequate counseling of patients regarding the disease process and what can be expected in the outpatient evaluation should also occur. It is important for the patient to understand that the hydatidiform mole, although evacuated during surgery, can recur and that her serum β-hCG levels will be carefully followed to assess for persistent or recurrent disease.

In order for the clinician to effectively manage a patient in the outpatient setting, future pregnancies must be prevented for at least 1 year or until cleared by the physician. So it is extremely important that each patient have a reliable form of contraception, preferably prior to hospital discharge. Most authorities also recommend obtaining a postevacuation chest radiograph and postevacuation β-hCG level within 48 hours. Follow-up should be scheduled with a physician who specializes in treating GTD, such as a gynecologic oncologist.

DISPOSITION
Discharge Goals

After the patient has demonstrated stability in the trend of postoperative hemoglobin and hematocrit values, the patient may successfully be discharged from the hospital with clear instructions about how the outpatient surveillance will proceed. In addition, it is extremely important that each patient have a reliable form of contraception prior to hospital discharge.

Outpatient Care

The outpatient management of postoperative molar pregnancies consists of prudent surveillance for recurrent, persistent, or malignant disease. To evaluate for malignant disease, one should review the inpatient chest radiographs. If they are negative for metastatic disease, studies have consistently found that one does not need to order further imaging to rule out other common areas of metastasis, such as the brain, the liver, and the kidneys.

However, some authorities recommend a full metastatic workup regardless of the chest radiograph results (1,2). The pathology report from the dilation and curettage should be reviewed, which helps to narrow down the diagnosis as to complete mole, partial mole, invasive mole, choriocarcinoma, or placental trophoblastic tumor. As stated earlier, these three previously mentioned forms of GTD, along with postmolar GTD, which is diagnosed by a plateau or an increase in serum β-hCG level, encompass gestational trophoblastic neoplasia. Risk factors for postmolar GTD are high pre-evacuation β-hCG levels, a uterine size greater than expected for the gestational age, theca-lutein cysts, and advanced maternal age. Serial pelvic exam while the β-hCG is elevated are also important to evaluate for potential vaginal metastases. The pathology report, the physical exam, and serial serum β-hCG measurements are vital tools to monitor patients for malignant GTD.

Serum β-hCG levels are obtained within 48 hours after evacuation, every 1 to 2 weeks while elevated, and then monthly for an additional six months. Criterion for diagnosing postmolar GTD by serum β-hCG levels was derived from consensus committee recommendations from the Society of Gynecologic Oncology, the International Gynecologic Cancer Society, and the International Society for the Study of Trophoblastic disease and proposed by the International Federation of Gynecologists and Obstetricians (FIGO). The criteria for postmolar GTD are a β-hCG level plateau of four values plus or minus 10% recorded over a 3-week period (days 1, 7, 14, and 21), a β-hCG level increase >10% of three values recorded over a 2-week period (days 1, 7, and 14), and/or persistent detectable β-hCG for more than 6 months after evacuation.

All patients with a pathologic diagnosis of choriocarcinoma, placental site trophoblastic tumor, or invasive mole require postevacuation chemotherapy. Chemotherapy is also initiated if metastatic disease is present or the serum β-hCG is plateauing or rising according to the aforementioned criteria. Prior to chemotherapy the clinician will classify the patient based on stage and low-risk versus high-risk disease to predict the likelihood of single-agent chemotherapy failure necessitating a need for multiagent chemotherapy. Stage one is disease confined to the uterus. Stage two is disease confined to the genital structures but extends outside the uterus. Stage three is metastatic disease in the lungs. Sage four includes all other metastatic sites. The FIGO scoring system is used to classify the patients into low-risk versus high-risk disease (Table 30-2).

The total prognostic score is obtained by adding up the individual scores for each category. Total score of 0 to 6 is low risk, 7 and above equals high risk.

You then combine the FIGO scoring and the FIGO clinical stage to determine the patient's treatment plan. For low-risk, nonmetastatic disease and low-risk metastatic GTD, single-agent chemotherapy with methotrexate or dactinomycin is used. Patients with high-risk metastatic disease will

TABLE 30-2

The International Federation of Gynecologists and Obstetricians (FIGO) Scoring System for Risk Assessment

FIGO Score	Age (years)	Antecedent Pregnancy	Interval from Index Pregnancy (months)	Pretreatment β-hCG (mIU/mL)	Largest Tumor Size (including uterus size, cm)	Site of Metastases	No. of Metastases	Previous Failed Chemotherapy
0	39	Hydatidiform mole	<4	<1,000	—	—	0	—
1	>39	Abortion	4–6	1,000–10,000	3–4	Spleen or kidney	1–4	—
2	—	—	6–12	10,000–100,000	5	Gastrointestinal system	4–8	Single drug
4	—	Term pregnancy	>12	>100,000	—	Brain or liver	>8	More than two drugs

β-hCG, beta–human chorionic gonadotropin.

be offered multiagent chemotherapy such as etoposide, methotrexate, dactinomycin, cyclophosphamide, and vincristine. For patients with placental site trophoblastic disease, hysterectomy is recommended because it is usually resistant to chemotherapy.

WHAT YOU NEED TO REMEMBER

- Gestational trophoblastic disease is a disease process of the placenta and encompasses many different individual disorders, including hydatidiform moles, choriocarcinoma, and placental site trophoblastic tumors.
- Complete moles are derived exclusively from paternal origin and are diploid, while partial moles have maternal and paternal genetic origins and are generally triploid.
- Medical complications, including acute blood loss anemia, early severe pre-eclampsia, hyperthyroidism, and coagulopathies, are important to recognize and stabilize prior to surgical management.
- The two surgical options for the management of the hydatidiform mole are dilation and curettage or hysterectomy.
- Serial serum β-hCG measurements, the physical exam, and selected imaging for evaluating metastatic disease should be part of outpatient management.
- If the serum β-hCG is plateauing or rising, metastatic disease is present, or the pathologic diagnosis of an invasive mole or a choriocarcinoma is suspected, patients will need chemotherapy.
- Single-agent chemotherapy is initiated for nonmetastatic and low-risk metastatic disease, while multiagent chemotherapy is used for high-risk metastatic disease.
- In the case of placental site trophoblastic disease, hysterectomy is the primary management.
- Patients should have a reliable method of contraception while undergoing treatment or the surveillance of GTD to prevent confusion in the management plan.

REFERENCES

1. DiSaia D, Creasman W. *Clinical Gynecologic Oncology.* 7th ed. St. Louis, MO: Mosby; 2007.
2. Kavanagh J, Gershenson D. Gestational trophoblastic disease: hydatidiform mole, nonmetastatic and metastatic gestational trophoblastic tumor. diagnosis and management. In: Katz VL, Lentz GM, Lobo RA, et al., eds. *Comprehensive Gynecology.* 5th ed. Philadelphia: Mosby Elsevier; 2007:889–901.

SUGGESTED READINGS

American College of Obstetricians and Gynecologists. ACOG practice bulletin number 53: diagnosis and treatment of gestational trophoblastic disease. *Obstet Gynecol.* 2004;103:1365–1377.

American College of Obstetricians and Gynecologists. *Compendium of Selected Publications.* Washington, DC: American College of Obstetricians and Gynecologists; 2007.

Sebire NJ, Seckl MJ. Gestational trophoblastic disease: current management of hydatidiform mole. *BMJ.* 2008;337:a1193.

Antepartum Fetal Assessment

In higher-risk pregnancies, there are times when testing the fetus for well-being will allow you to prolong the pregnancy and reduce the risks of prematurity. Presented here are the three most common tests used for antepartum fetal assessment: (i) NST (nonstress test), (ii) CST (contraction stress test), and (ii) BPP (biophysical profile).

NST (NONSTRESS TEST)

Reactive = two accelerations (15 beats per minute over baseline × 15 seconds) in 20 minutes (Fig. A1-1).

CST (CONTRACTION STRESS TEST)

Three contractions in a 10-minute period

Negative = no late decelerations.
Positive = late decelerations occurring with >50% of contractions.
Suspicious = any late decelerations.
Uterine hyperstimulation: contractions lasting >2 minutes and/or more than five contractions in 10 minutes

BPP (BIOPHYSICAL PROFILE)

Scoring system to evaluate fetal well-being (requires ultrasound)

Fetal breathing: one episode lasting >30 seconds in a 30-minute period = 2 points
Gross body movement: at least three body/limb movements in 30 minutes = 2 points
Fetal tone: one episode of active extension with return to flexion of fetal limbs/trunk in 30 minutes = 2 points
Reactive NST = 2 points
Amniotic fluid index (AFI): one pocket >2 cm in two perpendicular planes or AFI >8 = 2 points
Modified BPP = AFI + NST
Score each category with a 0 (abnormal) or a 2 (normal)
A score of >8 with normal AFI = reassuring
Any score >6 and/or decreased AFI = nonreassuring

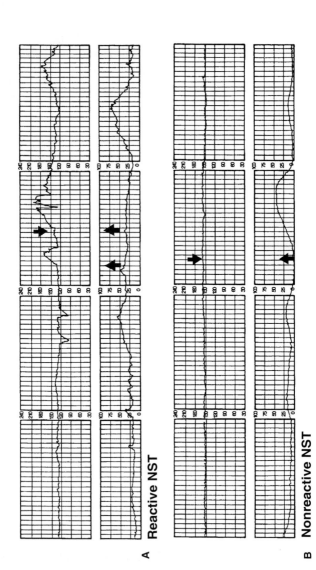

A Reactive NST

B Nonreactive NST

Electronic Fetal Monitoring

APPENDIX

2

Nearly 85% of all live births in the United States are evaluated using electronic fetal monitoring.[1] Despite the differences in the interpretation of electronic fetal monitoring among observers, there are clear pattern definitions and descriptions developed by the National Institute of Child Health and Human Development Working Group (Fig. A2-1).

EARLY DECELERATIONS

- A gradual decrease in the fetal heart rate when the nadir occurs at the same time as the peak of the contraction.
- Usually symmetrical and returns to baseline at the conclusion of the contraction.
- Usually related to a vagal response from head compression and does not indicate fetal hypoxia.

VARIABLE DECELERATIONS

- An abrupt decrease in the fetal heart rate.
- The decrease is >15 beats per minute, lasting between 15 and 120 seconds.
- The fetal heart rate reaches the nadir in <30 seconds.
- Usually related to umbilical cord compression.

LATE DECELERATIONS

- A gradual decrease in the fetal heart rate when the nadir occurs after the peak of the contraction.
- Usually caused by uteroplacental insufficiency.

REFERENCE

1. American College of Obstetricians and Gynecologists. ACOG practice bulletin number 70: intrapartum fetal heart rate monitoring. *Obstet Gynecol*. 2005;106: 1453–1461.

SUGGESTED READINGS

Macones GA, Hankins GDV, Spong CY, et al. The 2008 National Institute of Child Health and Human Development Workshop report on electronic fetal monitoring. Update on definitions, interpretation, and research guidelines. *Obstet Gynecol*. 2008;112:661–666.

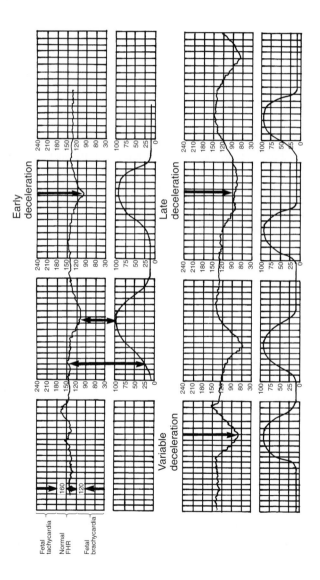

Early deceleration

Late deceleration

Variable deceleration

Fetal tachycardia

Normal FHR

Fetal brachycardia

160

120

Staging for Gynecologic Cancers

TABLE A3-1
Staging of Carcinoma of the Cervix Uteri

FIGO Stages		TNM Categories
	Primary tumor cannot be assessed	TX
	No evidence of primary tumor	T0
0	Carcinoma in situ (preinvasive carcinoma)	Tis
I	Cervical carcinoma confined to uterus (extension to corpus should be disregarded)	T1
IA	Invasive carcinoma diagnosed only by microscopy. All macroscopically visible lesions—even with superficial invasion—are Stage IB/T1b	T1a
IA1	Stromal invasion no greater than 3.0 mm in depth and 7.0 mm or less in horizontal spread	T1a1
IA2	Stromal invasion more than 3.0 mm and not more than 5.0 mm with a horizontal spread 7.0 mm or less^a	T1a2
IB	Clinically visible lesion confined to the cervix or microscopic lesion greater than IA2/T1a2	T1b
IB1	Clinically visible lesion 4.0 cm or less in greatest dimension	T1b1
IB2	Clinically visible lesion more than 4 cm in greatest dimension	T1b2
II	Turmour invades beyond the uterus but not to pelvic wall or to lower third of the vagina	T2
IIA	Without parametrial invasion	T2a
IIB	With parametrial invasion	T2b
III	Turmour extends to pelvic wall and/or involves lower third of vagina and/or causes hydronephrosis or nonfunctioning kidney	T3

(continued)

TABLE A3-1
Staging of Carcinoma of the Cervix Uteri (Continued)

FIGO Stages		TNM Categories
IIIA	Tumor involves lower third of vagina no extension to pelvic wall	T3a
IIIB	Tumor extends to pelvic wall and/or causes hydronephrosis or nonfunctioning kidney	T3b
IVA	Tumor invades mucosa of bladder or rectum and/or extends beyond true pelvis[b]	T4
IVB	Distand metastasis	M1

[a]*Note:* The depth of invasion should not be more than 5 mm taken from the base of the epithelium, either surface or glandular, from which it originates. The depth of invasion is defined as the measurement of the tumor from the epithelial-stromal junction of the adjacent most superficial epithelial papilla to the deepest point of invasion. Vascular space involvement, venous or lymphatic, does not affect classification.

[b]*Note:* The presence of bullous oedema is not sufficient to classify a tumor as T4.

TABLE A3-2

Carcinoma of the Corpus Uteri—Staging

FIGO Stages		TNM Categories
	Primary tumor cannot be assessed	TX
	No evidence of primary tumor	T0
0	Carcinoma in situ (preinvasive carcinoma	Tis
I	Tumor confined to the corpus uteri	T1
IA	Tumor limited to endometrium	T1a
IB	Tumor invades up to less than half of myometrium	T1b
IC	Tumor invades to more than one half of myometrium	T1c
II	Tumor invades cervix but does not extend beyond uterus	T2
IIA	Endocervical glandular involvement only	T2a
IIB	Cervical stromal invasion	T2b
III	Local and/or regional spread as specified in IIIA, B, C	T3 and/or N1
IIIA	Tumor involves serosa and/or adnexae (direct extension or metastasis) and/or cancer cells in ascites or peritoneal washings	T3a
IIIB	Vaginal involvement (direct extension or metastasis)	T3b
IIIC	Metastasis to pelvic and/or para-aortic lymph nodes	N1
IVA	Tumor invades bladder mucosa and/or bower mucosaa	T4
IVB	Distant metastasis (excluding metastasis to vagina, pelvic serosa, or adnexa, including metastasis to intra-abdominal lymph nodes other than para-aortic and/or inguinal nodes)	M1

Note: The presence of bullous oedema is not sufficient evidence to classify a tumor as T4.

TABLE A3-3

Staging of Carcinoma of the Ovary

FIGO			TNM
		Primary tumor cannot be assessed	TX
0		No evidence of primary tumor	T0
I		Tumor confined to ovaries	T1
	IA	Tumor limited to one ovary, capsule intact	T1a
		No tumor on ovarian surface	
		No malignant cells in the ascites or peritoneal washings	
	IB	Tumor limited to both ovaries, capsules intact	T1b
		No tumor on ovarian surface	
		No malignant cells in the ascites or peritoneal washings	
	IC	Tumor limited to one or both ovaries, with any of the following:	T1c
		Capsule ruptured, tumor on ovarian surface, positive malignant cells in the ascites or positive peritoneal washings	
II		Tumor involves one or both ovaries with pelvic extension	T2
	IIA	Extension and/or implants in uterus and/or tubes	T2a
		No malignant cells in the ascites or peritoneal washings	
	IIB	Extension to other pelvic organ	T2b
		No malignant cells in the ascites or peritoneal washings	
	IIC	IIA/B with positive malignant cells in the ascites or positive peritoneal washings	T2c

TABLE A3-3
Staging of Carcinoma of the Ovary (Continued)

FIGO		TNM
III	Tumor involves one or both ovaries with microscopically confirmed peritoneal metastasis outside the pelvis and/or regional lymph nodes metastasis	T3 and/or N1
IIIA	Microscopic peritoneal metastasis beyond the pelvis	T3a
IIIB	Macroscopic peritoneal metastasis beyond the pelvis 2 cm or less in greatest dimension	T3b
IIIC	Peritoneal metastasis beyond pelvis more than 2 cm in greatest dimension and/or regional lymph nodes metastasis	T3c and/or N1
IV	Distant metastasis beyond the peritoneal cavity	M1

Note: Liver capsule metastasis is T3/Stage III, liver parenchymal metastasis M1/stage IV. Pleural effusion must have positive cytology.

Index

Page numbers followed by f denote figure; page numbers followed by t denote table.

Growth restriction, intrauterine
    in diabetic mother with poor glycemic
        control, 3
    with hypertension, 2, 3
    with hypotension, 3
    preterm labor with, 51, 52t, 56
    from uteroplacental insufficiency, 3
Gynecologic cancer staging, 291t–295t
    for carcinoma of the cervix uteri, 291t–292t
    for carcinoma of the corpus uteri, 293t
    for carcinoma of the ovary, 294t–295t

H

Heart rate, fetal
    abnormalities of, 20–21
    assessment of, 10, 11t–12t, 13f
    electronic monitoring of, 11f, 289, 290f
    in labor and delivery, 10, 11t–12t, 13f, 15,
        18
    normal baseline, 15
    patterns of, 10, 11t–12t, 13f
HELLP syndrome, 47. See also Pre-eclampsia and
        eclampsia
    diagnosis of, 44, 45t
    disposition in, 48
    symptoms of, 46
Hemabate, reactive airway disease and, 69
Hemoglobin A1C
    for gestational diabetes diagnosis, 28
    prepregnancy target for, 4
Hemorrhage, postpartum. See Postpartum
        hemorrhage
Herpes simplex virus infection, genital
    history in, 140t–141t, 142
    treatment of, 146t, 147
Hidradenitis suppurativa, vulvar, 152t. See also
        Vulvar lesions
High-grade squamous intraepithelial lesion
        (HSIL), 257
Hormone replacement therapy (HR), for
        menopause, 234–235
Hot tubs, on male fertility, 219
Human menopausal gonadotropin (HMG), for
        unexplained infertility, 226t
Human papillomavirus (HPV)
    in cervical cancer, 254–255
    testing for, 257, 258
Human papillomavirus (HPV) vaccine, 261
Hydatidiform mole, 277–285
    acute management and workup of, 279–282
        first 15 minutes in, 279–280
        first few hours in, 280–282
            history and physical examination in,
                280
            labs and tests in, 280–281
            treatment in, 281–282
    definition of, 277
    disposition in, 282–285, 284t
    epidemiology of, 279
    etiology of, 279
    extended in-hospital management of, 282
    FIGO scoring system for, 283, 284t
    molar pregnancy features in, 278, 278t
Hydralazine, for severe hypertension in
        pregnancy, 44
17α-Hydroxyprogesterone, in female fertility, 221

Hyperglycemia, severe, in pregnancy, 27–28, 27t.
        See also Gestational diabetes (GDM)
Hypergonadotropic hypogonadism, 211t, 213,
        224
Hypermobile urethra, 249
Hyperprolactinemia, 191
Hypertension
    chronic
        methergine and, 69
        pre-eclampsia superimposed on, 42
        on pregnancy, 2–3, 2t
    gestational, 42
        definition of, 42
        diagnosis of, 44, 45t
    in pregnancy, 42 (See also Pre-eclampsia and
        eclampsia)
Hypertensive disorders of pregnancy. See Pre-
        eclampsia and eclampsia
Hypogastric artery ligation, for postpartum
        hemorrhage, 72, 74f
Hypoglycemia
    in gestational diabetes, 29, 31
    neonatal, 3
Hypogonadotropic hypogonadism, 211t,
        213–214, 224
Hypothalamic-pituitary-adrenal (HPA) axis
        activation, in preterm labor, 50
Hysterectomy
    for abnormal uterine bleeding, 177
    for cervical cancer, 260, 261
    for endometrial cancer, 274
    for hydatidiform mole, 281, 285
    for hypertension, 3
    for pelvic organ prolapse, 237
    pelvic relaxation after, 237
    for postpartum hemorrhage, 73

I

Ileal conduit urinary diversion, for urinary
        incontinence, 251
Implanon, 104
Implantable contraception, 104
Incomplete abortion, 127, 128t, 129f
Incontinence, urinary, 245–252
    acute management and workup of, 247–251
        first 15 minutes in, 247
        first few hours in, 248–251
            history in, 248
            labs and tests in, 249–250
            physical examination in, 248–249
            treatment in, 250–251
    definition of, 245
    disposition in, 252
    epidemiology of, 245–246
    etiology of, 246–247
    extended in-hospital management of, 252
    overflow, 246
    pathophysiology of, 245
    stress, 246
    urge, 246
Indomethacin, for preterm labor, 56–57
Inevitable abortion, 127, 128t
Infection, genital. See also specific infections
    postpartum fever from, 78t, 84t (See also
        Postpartum fever)
    in preterm labor, 50–51